The Benefits of Homoeopathy

The Benefits of

Homoeopathy

Vijaya Kumar

NEW DAWN PRESS, INC.
USA• UK• INDIA

NEW DAWN PRESS GROUP

Published by New Dawn Press Group
New Dawn Press, Inc., 244 South Randall Rd # 90, Elgin, IL 60123
e-mail: sales@newdawnpress.com

New Dawn Press, 2 Tintern Close, Slough, Berkshire, SL1-2TB, UK
e-mail: sterlingdis@yahoo.co.uk

New Dawn Press (An Imprint of Sterling Publishers (P) Ltd.)
A-59, Okhla Industrial Area, Phase-II, New Delhi-110020
e-mail: sterlingpublishers@airtelbroadband.in
www.sterlingpublishers.com

The Benefits of Homoeopathy
© 2006, by Vijaya Kumar
ISBN 1 84557 626 8

PRINTED IN INDIA

Preface

Homoeopathy is a holistic and complete scientific system of medicine. It has been in worldwide use for nearly two hundred years. People suffering from all kinds of illnesses, from depression to arthritis, migraine to ulcers, cancers to more modern illnesses like AIDS and myalgic encephalomyelitis, can be helped by homoeopathy to regain their health.

Most importantly, since homoeopathy medicines are in dilutions, the side effects are grossly minimised. Hence, this system is perfect in ailments of infants and children.

A good remedy removes the disease from its roots and leaves no trace of the disease behind. A person's constitution is given prime importance in homoeopathy because no two individuals are alike. Hence, we have one drug per individual, and this path thus becomes unique and more accurate. Case taking is the most vital part prior to treatment wherein the mental symptoms along with the physical are analysed by the doctors. There is a concept of vital force and miasms which determine the health status and a person's future health condition which are again unique to the principle of this path.

Homoeopathy has made tremendous advance, with pioneers such as Dr. Samuel Hahnemann, Dr. James Tyler Kent, Dr. Boeninghausen, Dr. Boericke, and so on, making voluminous contributions and enhancing the spread of this branch the world over. It is recognised internationally as a branch of complementary and alternative medicine.

Homoeopathy in India enjoys government support along with the other systems of medicine because government is of the view that the presence of all these complementary alternative systems of therapeutics offers a much wider spectrum of curative medicine than is available in any other country.

The information contained in this book is for education, not the practice of medicine.

Contents

1

Introduction

'Homoeopathy' is derived from the Greek words *homoeos* (like or similar) and *pathos* (disease or suffering), which means 'likes cure likes'. The efficacy of homoeopathy drugs is well-established in almost all the ailments, including those which are a challenge to the modern medicine, such as rheumatoid, arthritis, cancer, diabetes mellitus, etc.

Homoeopathy was discovered by Dr. Samuel Hahnemann, a German physician, in 1790. During one of his experiments he noticed that ingesting the juice of the bark of cinchona, he developed malarial symptoms, like chills, fever, nausea, whereas cinchona drug was actually used to treat malaria. Thus, a new system of medicine evolved, called homoeopathy, based on the principle 'Similia Similibus Curantur', which means 'likes cure likes'. That is, a drug that produces a certain set of symptoms in a healthy individual can cure the same in a diseased individual.

In his experiments, Dr Hahnemann developed a method of 'potentising' homoeopathic remedies by diluting them in a water alcohol solution, and then vigorously shaking (or succussing) the mixtures. The results convinced him that a high degree of dilution not only minimises the side effects of the remedies but also simultaneously enhances their medicinal powers.

Over the past two decades, the use of homoeopathic remedies and visits to homoeopathic practitioners have increased. One possible reason reported is clinical efficacy. Some homoeopathic patients may have personally found previous treatment to be effective or heard from friends, colleagues, and the media, of many cases in which a sickness was healed after homoeopathic treatment. Some reinforce their favourable judgement with selective reference to positive scientific reports. Though they are aware that science has found no adequate explanation for the mechanism of homoeopathy, they may subscribe to an empirical view of the matter. Whatever works in their experience is good enough for them. This attitude arguably characterises most health consumers nowadays, whose main concern is for perceived efficacy rather than scientific sanction for their choice of treatment. This attraction is possibly further amplified from the inability by conventional health care to treat long-term diseases.

Another reason could be dissatisfaction with allopathic treatment. Some reject the medical establishment, which is perceived to place too much emphasis on machines and chemicals, and to treat the disease, not the person. Homoeopathic practitioners often spend more time dealing with their patients than conventional practitioners. Furthermore, homoeopathic preparations have few, if any, side effects, and are generally much cheaper than conventional medications.

Some are attracted to homoeopathy through its holistic worldview, their desire for their story to be heard out in detail, their belief that their individually diagnosed complaints belong together in one pattern, and so on.

There is a holistic as well as individualistic approach to medicine through homoeopathy. This is a key point, and unique to homoeopathy. Even though it may sound strange, homoeopathy does not treat disease per se. A homoeopath does not concentrate his therapy on, say arthritis or bronchitis or cancer. In other words, he does not limit his treatment to painful joints, inflamed bronchi or a malignant growth. Rather, he treats all aspects – mental, emotional and physical – of the person who happens to be suffering from arthritis or bronchitis or cancer. Homoeopathy regards each patient' as a unique individual. For example, six persons with hepatitis might get a different homoeopathic remedy, each one aimed at the individual's totality of symptoms rather than at his liver alone. The physician's interest is not only to alleviate the patients' present symptoms but also their long-term well-being.

Homoeopathy is based on certain fixed laws and principles that are as true and as unchanged today as the law of gravity. These include the Law of Similars, the minimum dose, the single remedy, the vital force, the chronic miasms, the law of direction of cure, and so on.

The science of homoeopathic medicine is based on ascertained facts and abundantly proved deductions. Right from the process of proving of drugs to the prescription of the curative remedy, the methods are controlled by the principles of inductive reasoning.

In *Principles and Practice of Homoeopathy,* Dr. M.L. Dhawle states,

> "Hahnemann was the first clinician to exploit fully the language of symptoms for diagnostic as well as therapeutic purposes. He was the first clinician to work out scientifically the curative relationship between the effects of disease and the effects of drugs. Prior to him, therapeutics was based on dogma and empiricism which led to all types of irrational and often harmful practices."

Homoeopathy is the medicine of vital stimulation of mind, which directs all aspects of life in the organism. Disease, as viewed by homoeopathy, is a dynamic expression of the disturbances of the harmony and rhythm of the vital force. The defence mechanism acting on all three levels of the organism (mental, emotional, physical), is the tool of the vital force acting in the context of the disease. Without the vital force the whole body becomes inanimate and sick.

Prevention, care and maintenance are best done by behaviour modification, dietary regulation and, where permissible, a regular exercise regimen. Herbal medicines and vitamins may help.

The study of homoeopathy is valuable for all those who wish to understand the laws of nature, the principles of healing and the meaning of health and disease of all the branches of medicine. Homoeopathy is most closely related to the laws of nature and human nature.

What is Homoeopathy?

Homoeopathy is one of the scientific systems of medicine based on the principle, '*Similia Similibus Curantur*', meaning 'likes cure likes'. This concept is similar to the 'Samam Samenah Shanthi' concept of Indian thought. Homoeopathy is an effective system of healing which assists the natural tendency of the body to heal itself.

Homoeopathy is an alternative medical system. Alternative medical systems are built upon complete systems of theory and practice, and often have evolved apart from and earlier than the conventional medical approach used in many parts of the world. Homoeopathy takes a different approach from conventional medicine in diagnosing, classifying and treating medical problems.

The homoeopathic system of holistic healing was founded by Dr. Samuel Hahnemann, a German physician. While translating a book on the medicinal properties of drugs, he read about the properties of the healing powers of the bark of the cinchona tree. Due to its bitter taste, cinchona was said to cure malaria. This set him thinking, and he decided to test the medicine on himself, after reading a footnote which stated that cinchona poisoning leads to malaria-like symptoms. He experienced the symptoms of malaria, by repeatedly taking the cinchona medicine. He found that those medicines which cause disease-like symptoms in healthy individuals are capable of curing the diseased individuals. So homoeopathy relies on the *Materia Medica,* a book containing the properties of medicines, which have been proved on healthy individuals.

Homoeopathy: A Holistic System

Homoeopathy is considered to be holistic medicine also. The holistic approach to medicine takes a wider view of illness, a wider view of the causes of disease and the ways in which people express their illness individually. It claims to provoke healing responses to diseases by administering specially prepared substances that mimic the symptoms of those diseases in healthy people. It recognises that all symptoms of ill health are expressions of disharmony within the whole person, and that it is the patient who needs treatment, not the disease.

Homocopathy is holistic because it treats the whole person, and its remedies assist people to regain health by stimulating their natural healing forces. Homoeopaths treat physical, emotional, mental and even the spiritual aspects of each patient, since homoeopaths regard these areas as being intimately connected, and all part of the whole of the patient's suffering.

Law of Similars

Homoeopathic remedies and treatments are tailored specifically to the needs of the individual and not just their disease or illness – for the person's whole state at that time. Like Hippocrates two thousand years earlier, Samuel Hahnemann realised that there are two ways of treating ill health – the way of opposites and the way of similars. Take, for example, a case of insomnia. The way of opposites (conventional medicine or allopathy) is to treat this by giving a drug to bring on an artificial sleep. This frequently involves the use of large or regular dose of drugs which can sometimes cause side effects or addiction.

The way of similars, the homoeopathic way, is to give the patient a minute dose of a substance, such as tea or coffee, which in large doses causes sleeplessness in a healthy person. Perhaps, surprisingly, this will enable the patient to sleep naturally.

Two patients with apparently similar illnesses may be treated with different remedies. The homoeopath is interested in matters which may seem to have little or nothing to do with the complaint that the patient is more concerned with, but contributes to the person's total well-being.

Concepts of Homoeopathy

The key concepts of homoeopathy include:

1. Homoeopathy seeks to stimulate the body's defence mechanisms and processes so as to prevent or treat illness.
2. Treatment involves giving very small doses of substances called remedies that, according to homoeopathy, would produce the same or similar symptoms of illness in healthy people if they were given in larger doses.
3. Treatment in homoeopathy is individualised, or tailored to each person. Homoeopathic practitioners select remedies according to a total picture of the patient, including not only symptoms but lifestyle, emotional and mental states, and other factors.

Homoeopathy has been serving suffering humanity for over two centuries, has withstood the upheavals of time, and has emerged as a time-tested therapy. The scientific principles propounded by Hahnemann are natural and well-proven, and continue to be followed with success.

Homoeopathy around the World

Samuel Hahnemann's Experiments

Around 1800, the German medical doctor, obviously appalled with the still mostly medieval medical practices of his contemporaries, set out to revolutionise medical science. He began developing the homoeopathic method after coming upon the idea that 'likes cure likes' while translating a work on malaria. Upon reaching a passage that 'quinine' (extracted from the bark of the cinchona tree) was an effective treatment because it was bitter and astringent, Hahnemann felt this implausible because there were many other substances that were equally bitter yet lacked any therapeutic value. To better understand the effects of quinine, he decided to take it himself, and observed that his reactions were similar to the symptoms of the disease it was used to treat.

For Hahnemann and his students the whole of the body and spirit was the focus of therapy, not just the localised disease. Hahnemann himself spent extended periods of time with his patients, asking them questions that dealt not only with their particular symptoms or illness, but also with the details of their daily lives. It is also suggested that the gentle approach of homoeopathy was a reaction to the violent forms of 'heroic medicine' common at the time which included techniques such as bleeding as a matter of course.

During a lifetime of hard and dedicated work, Hahnemann wrote several books and constructed the mainstay of what was to become homoeopathic medicines. His books and teachings still form the foundation and the main substance of homoeopathy today. Starting from sound chemical practice, he built a complete system of natural laws and an extensive pharmacopoeia of homoeopathic medicines.

When Hahnemann began working as a physician, chemist and linguist in the late 1700's, it was a time when the most common medical treatments were harsh, such as purging, blistering, bleeding, and the use of sulphur and mercury. Hence, he was determined to develop a less-threatening approach to medicine. His principle of 'Similia Similibus Curantur' has a prior history in medicine from Hippocrates in Ancient Greece – who noted, for example, that recurrent vomiting could be treated with an emetic, such as ipecacuanha, that would be expected to make it worse – to folk medicine. Hahnemann's view that 'likes cure likes' was that symptoms are part of the body's response to an infection, and a cough may help to eliminate mucus – and medication may be given to support this self-healing response.

Hahnemann tested single, pure substances on himself and, in more dilute forms, on healthy volunteers. He kept meticulous records of his experiments and participants' responses, and he combined these observations with the information from clinical practice, the known uses of herbs and other medicinal substances, and toxicology, eventually treating the sick and developing homoeopathic clinical practice.

Hahnemann added two additional elements to homoeopathy:

1. A concept that became 'potentiation', which holds that systematically diluting a substance, with vigorous shaking at each step of dilution, makes the remedy more, not less, effective by extracting the vital essence of the substance. If the dilution comes to the point where the substance's molecules are gone, homoeopathy holds that the effects they exerted on the surrounding water molecules may still be therapeutic.

2. A concept that treatment should be selected based upon a total picture of an individual and his symptoms, not solely upon symptoms of a disease. Homoeopaths evaluate not only a

person's physical symptoms but his emotional and mental states, lifestyle, nutrition and other aspects. In homoeopathy, different people with the same symptoms may receive different homoeopathic remedies.

The World Health Organisation noted in 1994 that homoeopathy had been integrated into the national health care systems of numerous countries including Germany, the United Kingdom, India, Pakistan, Sri Lanka and Mexico.

Homoeopathy in India

Homoeopathy was brought to the Indian medical system when Maharaja Ranjit Singh, the ruler of Punjab, summoned Dr. John Martin Honigberger in 1839 to treat him for paralysis of vocal cords and oedema. After being completely cured, he made Dr. Honigberger officer-in-command of a hospital. Later, Dr. Honigberger established practice in Calcutta. This royal patronage helped homoeopathy to have its roots in India. Several missionaries and amateurs in Indian civil and military service practised homoeopathy extensively, and spread this system in West Bengal and South India.

Soon after independence, the Government of India developed the homoeopathic system of medicine by setting up the Homoeopathic Enquiry Committee in 1948, the Planning Commission in 1951, and the Homoeopathic Pharmacopoeia Committee in 1962. At the recommendations of these committees, homoeopathy has been accepted by the government as one of the national systems of medicine. During the Second Five Year Plan, funds were released for its development. Some states encouraged education of homoeopathy and employment of homoeopaths in health services, and regulated the practice by enacting States Acts and Rules.

The Indian government established the Indian Systems of Medicine, and homoeopathy was assigned a key role in the delivery of primary health care. The National Health Policy passed by the government envisaged its integration in the overall health care delivery system, especially in the preventive and promotive aspects of health care in the context of the national target of achieving 'Health for All by AD 2000'.

By the beginning of the twentieth century, a number of homoeopathy dispensaries mushroomed in major cities in India. In 1973, on the recommendations of the various committees set up by the government, a Central Act was passed for recognition of homoeopathy as one of the national systems of medicine in India.

Homoeopathy today is a rapidly growing system in India. It has become a household name due to the safety of its pills and gentleness of its cure. A general study indicates that about 15 per cent of the Indian population solely depends on homoeopathy for its health care needs.

It is more than a century and a half now that homoeopathy is being practised in India. It has blended in so well into the roots and traditions of the country that it has been recognised as one of the national systems of education of medicine and provides the much needed gentle cure and health care to a large number of people. Its strength lies in its evident effectiveness as it takes a holistic approach towards the sick individual through promotion of inner balance at mental, emotional, spiritual and physical levels.

Homoeopathy in Europe

There are estimated to be over a lakh physicians practising homoeopathy worldwide, with an estimated 500 million people receiving treatment. Over 12,000 medical doctors and licensed health care homoeopaths administer treatment in the UK, France and Germany. The latest amendments to the directive passed by the European Union in 2001 make it mandatory for all member states to implement a special registration procedure for homoeopathic remedies.

Homoeopathy in US

Homoeopathy was introduced in the United States in 1825, and rapidly gained in popularity, partly due to the fact that the excesses of conventional medicine were especially extreme there, and partly due to the efforts of Constantine Hering. Homoeopathy reached its peak of popularity in America between 1865 and 1885, and thereafter, declined due to a combination of the recognition by the establishment of the dangers of large doses of drugs and bleeding, and dissent between different schools of homoeopathy.

Another person who (like Hahnemann) was responsible for the development and popularisation of homoeopathy was the American physician, James Tyler Kent (1849-1821). His most important contribution may be his repertory which is still widely used today. Kent's approach to homoeopathy was decidedly authoritarian emphasising the metaphysical and clinical aspects of Hahnemann's teachings, in particular:

1. insistence on the doctrines of miasm and vitalism.
2. more emphasis on psychological symptoms (as opposed to physical pathology), and
3. regular use of very high potencies.

Kent's influence in the US was somewhat limited, but his ideas were reintroduced in the UK, where they became the homoeopathic orthodoxy by the end of the First World War.

In the 1930's, the popularity of homoeopathy began to wane, especially in Europe and the United States, partly due to advances in biology and conventional medicines, and partly due to the Flexner Report in 1910 which led to the closure in North America, of virtually all medical schools teaching alternative medicine. Another reason was a decline in coherence in the homoeopathic community.

Homoeopathy experienced a renaissance in the 1970's, largely thanks to the efforts of George Vithoulkas in Europe and the United States, that continues to this day. In India, homoeopathy had remained relatively strong throughout the twentieth century due to its isolation from the above factors, and at present Indian homoeopaths are among the most influential worldwide. Finally, the rise in popularity of homoeopathy must also be seen as part of the general rise in interest in alternative medicine over the past few decades.

The ease with which large databases can be manipulated has brought about profound changes in the way homoeopathy is practised. Today, many homoeopaths use personal computers to sift through thousands of pages of provings and case studies. Since the information about lesser-known remedies is more accessible, it is now more common for homoeopaths to prescribe them, which in turn has led to an increase in the number of new provings. Database technology has also encouraged researchers to recognise and restructure existing information.

In the United States, homoeopathic remedies are, like all health care products, subject to regulation by the Food and Drug Administration. However, the FDA accords homoeopathic remedies a treatment significantly different from that accorded to other drugs. Homoeopathic products are not required to be approved by the FDA prior to sale, not required to be proven either safe or effective prior to being sold, not required to be labelled with an expiry date, and not required to undergo finished product testing to verify contents and strengths. Homoeopathic remedies have their own imprints that, unlike conventional drugs, do not have to identify their active ingredients on the grounds that they have few or no active ingredients. In the United States, only homoeopathic medicines that claim to treat self-limiting conditions may be sold over the counter, while homoeopathic medicines that claim to treat a serious disease can be sold only by prescription. Neither the American Medical Association nor the American Academy of Paediatrics has an official policy for or against homoeopathy. Homoeopathy's popularity in the United States is growing.

Homoeopathy in Germany

In Germany, more than six thousand physicians specialise in homoeopathy. In 1978, homoeopathy, along with anthroposophically extended medicine and herbatism, were recognised as 'special forms of therapy', meaning that their medications are free from the usual requirement of proving efficacy. Since January 1, 2004, homoeopathic medications, albeit with some exceptions, are no longer covered by the country's public health insurance. Most private health insurers continue to cover homoeopathy.

Homoeopathy in Austria

In Austria, homoeopathy has been recognised as part of the medical system since 1983.

Homoeopathy in Switzerland

In Switzerland, homoeopathy is one of the five classes of complementary medicine. At one time, homoeopathic medications were covered by the basic health insurance system, as long as they were prescribed by a physician. This practice ended in June 2005.

Homoeopathy in the UK

In the United Kingdom, as in most countries, homoeopathic medicines may be sold over the counters. The UK has five homoeopathic hospitals where treatment, funded by the National Health Service, is available, and there are numerous regional clinics. Homoeopathy is not practised by the majority of the medical profession but there is a core of public support, especially in Scotland and also from the English royal family. In fact, homoeopathy is called 'The Royal Medicine' because Britain's royal family has used it since the 1830's.

4

How Does Homoeopathy Work?

Within the limitations of available scientific funding, interesting research is being undertaken to understand how and why such highly diluted remedies have profound and curative effects. How these incredibly minute doses can have such resonance in our bodies is a little too technical for science quite yet, though science is finding more and more applications for energetically diluted substances in and out of the medicine from engine additives to experiments in chemotherapy.

How homoeopathic medicines work is presently a mystery. And yet, nature is replete with striking examples of the powerful effects of extremely small doses of active agents. It is commonly known that certain species of moths can smell pheromones of its own species up to two miles away. Likewise, sharks are known to sense blood in the water at large distances. Similarly, small doses of medicine will not have any effect unless the person is hypersensitive to the specific medicinal substance. Hypersensitivity is created when there is some type of resonance between the medicine and the person.

Law of Similars

Since the system of homoeopathy bases its selection of the medicine on its ability to cause in overdose the similar symptoms that the sick person is experiencing, homoeopathy's 'law of similars' is simply a practical method of finding the substance to which the person is hypersensitive.

The homoeopathic principle of similars makes further sense when one considers that physiologists and pathologists now recognise that disease is not simply the result of breakdown or surrender of the body but that symptoms are instead representative of the body's efforts to fight infection or adopt to stress. Fever, inflammation, pain, discharge, and even high blood pressure are but a small number of the common symptoms that the organism creates in order to defend and to try to heal itself.

After over 200 years of experience, homoeopathic physicians have found that a homoeopathic medicine acts longer and deeper when it is more potentised. Although no one knows precisely why this happens, it is conjectured that highly potentised small doses can more deeply penetrate cells and the blood brain barrier than less potentised medicines. Although there is no consensus on why these small doses work more deeply, there is consensus from users of these natural medicines that they do.

Vital Force

The theory behind the working of homoeopathy is that the body of every human being contains a vital force within the body which regulates the functioning of the body. Due to reasons such as heredity, environmental conditions, stress, etc., this vital force weakens, causing a disease which is nothing but a complex of certain symptoms observed in the human body. The homoeopath makes a study of not only the symptoms the patient is complaining of, but of the entire patient himself. Since all patients are unique, homoeopathic medicines are prescibed to treat patients as individuals. For example, headaches in different patients would be treated with different medicines, according to the patient's individual symptoms.

Potentiation

The preparation of homoeopathic medicines consists of repeated dilution and shaking called 'potentiation'. Homoeopaths believe this process renders the remedies capable of stimulating the body's natural healing forces. After the twelfth dilution, there is no discernible chemical trace of the original substance left in the medicine. Scientists question how this highly diluted substance could retain a biological effect, but homoeopaths believe the preparation retains the qualities of the original substance.

Our bodies have incredibly sensitive receptors which trigger adjustments and responses to even the slightest changes and dangers in our environment – changes, which, thanks to these receptors, we usually know nothing about. The body adjusts to every temperature change to chemicals in the air and in our food, to fluorescent lights, germs and bacteria present in every breath we take, it responds to bitterness, dryness, acidity, and so on. Only when these aggravants are in excess, or our reactions are too burdened, do we ever know what changes our systems have made to keep us comfortable and safe. This is not news to those of us who know the healing powers of homoeopath's extremely minute doses. In response to the slightest hint that something is present which can cause a certain set of symptoms, the body sets out to heal itself.

Formal studies published in current medical journals show that homoeopathic remedies, when used correctly, are significantly very effective. Researchers theorise that, during potentiation, an energetic change occurs in the remedy substance and its medium of dilution (usually water, or at times alcohol), enabling them to stimulate a person's system to deal with stress and illness more efficiently. Homoeopathic remedies do not have chemical action in the body, and thus work differently than nutrients or drugs – which has made it difficult for some researchers accustomed to accessing drugs to adequately consider them. Since the body is clearly affected by many forces that have no chemical content, it is reasonable to think that research designed to observe non-chemical effects will yield more useful information.

The basic idea of homoeopathy is that the human body's natural state is one of health, and that we possess the ability to heal ourselves. It is a belief based on the idea that symptoms are not meant to be suppressed with medication but used as an indication of what the body needs in order to heal itself. The idea is that when we follow the directions provided by our symptoms, we will know to stimulate our healing processes in order to make ourselves well.

Homoeopathic doctors dilute known medicines in order to make them more powerful, according to their beliefs, while minimising toxic reactions and negative side effects. They consider the well-being of the whole patient – mental, emotional and physical – when deciding upon a treatment whereas conventional doctors often only consider the physical manifestations of an illness and how to treat it.

According to most homoeopathic beliefs, homoeopathy utilises safe preparations of natural substances, about 80 per cent of which are derived from plants like wild hops (*Bryonia*), marigold (*Calendula*), and poison ivy (*Rhus toxicodendron*). Other remedies come from animals or animal products like honey and inky fluid from cuttlefish. Still other remedies come from minerals and mineral ores like sodium chloride, and sulphur.

Minimum Dose

Homoeopathic medicine presents a significantly different pharmacological approach to treating sick people. Instead of using strong and powerful doses of medicinal agents that have a broad-spectrum effect on a wide variety of people with a similar disease, homoeopaths use extremely small doses of medicinal substances that are highly individualised to a person's physical and psychological syndrome of disease, not simply an assumed localised pathology.

Homoeopathic medicines are so small in dose that it is appropriate to refer to them as a part of a newly defined field of nanopharmacology. To understand the nature and degree of homoeopathy's pharmacology, it is important to know the following characteristics of how homoeopathic medicines are made.

1. Most homoeopathic medicines are made by diluting a medicinal substance in a double distilled water. It should be noted that physicists who study the properties of water commonly

acknowledge that water has many mysterious properties. Since homoeopaths use a double-distilled water, it is highly purified, enabling the medicinal substance to solely infiltrate the water. The medicinal solution is usually preserved in an 87 per cent water-alcohol solution.

2. Each substance is diluted, most commonly, one part of the original medicinal agent to nine or 99 parts double-distilled water. The mixture is then vigorously stirred or shaken. The solution is then diluted again 1:9 or 1:99, and vigorously stirred. This process of diluting and stirring is repeated – 3, 6, 12, 20, 200, 1,000 or even 1,000,000 times.

3. It is inaccurate to say that homoeopathic medicines are just extremely diluted; they are extremely 'potentised'. Potentiation refers to the specific process of sequential dilution with vigorous stirring. The theory is that each consecutive dilution in conjunction with the process of shaking/stirring infiltrates the new double-distilled water, and imprints upon it the fractal form of the original substance used (fractal refers to the specific consecutively smaller pattern or form within a larger pattern).

Homoeopathic medicines are given in highly dilute doses so as to prevent side effects. These minute doses create a similar disorder in the vital force of the patient as in a healthy person, provoking the vital force to react to the symptoms and overcome them. The same system is used in vaccines, where vaccination against smallpox is done by injecting the patient with the smallpox disease-causing organism, so that the body can build up its natural immunity.

5

Principles and Philosophy

The principles of homoeopathy has been since the time of Hippocrates from Greece, the founder of medicine, around 450 BC. More than a thousand years later, the Swiss alchemist, Paracelsus, employed the same system of healing based upon the principle that 'likes cure likes'. But it was not until eighteenth century that homoeopathy, as it is practised today, was evolved by the great German physician, Dr. Samuel Hahnemann. He was appalled by the medical practices of that time, and set about to develop a method of healing which would be safe, gentle and effective. He believed that human beings have the capacity to heal themselves, and that the symptoms of disease reflect the individual's struggle to overcome his illness.

Dr. Hahnemann recorded his experiments in *The Organon,* the essence of which can be described as follows:

"The like remedy, the single drug, the smallest dose, the infrequent dose, non-interference with the organism's vital reactions, occasional initial and minor aggravation, and potentiation of the remedy.

"To cure mildly, rapidly and permanently, choose in every case of disease, a remedy which can itself produce a similar affection."

Law of Similars

Based on some practical observations and on logic, Hahnemann developed a theory which he called 'the law of similars'. According to this theory, a medicine that causes the same symptoms as those of the disease will override the disease, such that the morbid function of the vital force will be caused by the medicine, not the original disease, and as the effect of the medicine wears off, the patient will be left cured. Thus, Hahnemann declared the group of homoeopathic medicines to be the one and only path to cure.

To find out what symptoms various substances caused, Hahnemann used a purely empirical approach. He administered the substance to healthy persons (often himself) and carefully recorded the effects. This is called 'proving'. Thus, if a substance caused headache, it should be assumed to be able to cure headache. It is not as simple as that, however, because just as a disease is not viewed as a single symptom but as a complete symptom profile essentially unique to each case, the effect of a substance on a healthy person is rarely a single distinct symptom, but rather a set of symptoms. Hahnemann recorded anything that the test subject felt during testing as caused by the medical substance, unless it was very evidently something the person had also been experiencing prior to the proving.

According to him, the primary principle underlying homoeopathy is 'Similia Similibus Curantur'—let like be cured by like. A symptom or pattern of symptoms can be healed by a substance in nature which can cause those symptoms. In other words, by finding the substance in nature which can cause the same conditions we are experiencing, we can give a dose so dilute that it is absolutely safe and still gives our bodies just the formulae they need to stimulate many levels of cure.

Hahnemann was struck by the effect that certain drugs, when taken by him while quite healthy, produced symptoms that the drug was known to cure in a sick. He wondered if the reason cinchona worked against intermittent fever was because it caused symptoms indistinguishable from intermittent fever in a healthy human.

He continued to experiment, noting that every substance he took, whether a herb, a mineral, an animal product or a chemical compound, produced definite distinct symptoms in him. He further noted that no substances produced exactly the same set of symptoms. Each provoked its own unique pattern of symptoms. Furthermore, the symptoms were not just confined to the physical plane. Every substance tested also affected the mind and the emotions apart from the body. Eventually, Hahnemann began to treat the sick on the principle 'Let likes be treated by likes'. From the outset he achieved outstanding clinical success.

Simplex, Similimum, Minimum

The principle of '*Simplex, Similimum, Minimum*' consists of three words. The first is 'Simplex', simple medicines, not compound, should be prescribed. This is the doctrine of single remedy. Mixture of medicines or polypharmacy is not allowed. Only one, a single medicine must be given at a time. '*Similimum*' means, when the totality of symptoms of the patient is taken, it will yield a picture which corresponds to one medicine, the *similimum,* which must be given. That medicine which has been tested on various people and has produced similar symptoms as that of the patient is the similar remedy. 'Minimum' means a low dosage of medicine is recommended. In homoeopathy, *less is more,* so medicines of low potency and given at long intervals have a better impact. Hahnemann, in fact, used to give just one dose of the medicine and wait to see the reaction over a period of time.

In evaluating the need to repeat or change a remedy, the single drug gives the best indication of which direction to take. The key word to remember is wait. Allow the remedy to find its own level of resonance, regardless of time.

With an acute illness, often, improvement can be seen within four to eight hours after the first dose, sometimes even sooner. If there is no effect or change, then another remedy can be considered.

The first question which confronts is, whether to give one dose or repeated doses. The second question is, if we give one dose, when shall we repeat it? Third, if we give repeated doses, how often shall we repeat the doses, and when shall we stop dosing?

Many physicians start with a single dose of the indicated remedy and await reaction. The duration of action of a remedy which acts varies, of course, with the nature and rate of progress of the disease. In a disease that worsens quickly towards death, like cholera, the action of the indicated remedy might be exhausted in five or ten minutes, and another dose be required soon after. In a slowly progressing disease like tuberculosis, the action of a dose of a curative remedy might continue for two or three months. Between these two extremes are all degrees of variation. The only rule which can be laid down with safety is to repeat the dose only when improvement ceases.

In homoeopathy, only one remedy is used at a time. Just as a television reproduces only the programme to which it is tuned, so a sick person is very sensitive to or 'tuned-in' to, the correct remedy, and only a minute stimulus, from the right signal (or remedy) is required. This is sometimes called the principle of minimum dose. The idea is to cure with the minimum amount of medicine and the minimum of intervention.

It is the body's energy which is influenced rather than its chemical balance, and the remedies do not cause side effects, as there is no chemical trace to accumulate in the body's tissues. For the same reason it is not possible to take an overdose of homoeopathic medicine in the same way as in orthodox medicine (orthodox medicine works on a chemical level).

Homoeopathic medicines are not therefore intrinsically dangerous. None the less, they are clearly capable of stimulating the body's reactive forces powerfully, and should be treated with respect.

The principle of minimum dose states that extreme dilution enhances the curative properties of a substance, while eliminating any possible side effects. This is just the reverse of conventional drug philosophy where concentration of the drug is effective.

Vital Force

Non-interference with the organism's vital reactions embodies Hahnemann's ideas on the vital force. This vital force is said to be the difference between a living and a dead thing (although Hahnemann does not quite equate it to a soul), and it is assumed to be the superior regulator of health. At Hahnemann's time, the very limited knowledge of the functioning of the body left ample space for surmising such a force. The basic principle of homoeopathy is based on the functioning of this vital force which is described as a non-materialistic property of all living creatures. If the vital force is functioning well, the creature is healthy; if not, the creature becomes ill. Disease is defined as a unique set of symptoms characteristic of the particular condition of the particular patient. Homoeopathy only recognises causes of disease as disturbing agents for the vital force, and distinct diseases only as categories of cases that display similar symptom profiles. Hahnemann specifically discouraged looking for hidden causes and diagnosing diseases per name.

To cure, one needs medicines, and as homoeopathy basically only recognises symptoms, which are interpreted then as disturbances in the functioning of the vital force, it follows logically that medicines must be substances that are somehow able to affect the vital force, causing some kind of symptoms to emerge.

Elaborating on this train of logic, Hahnemann divided medicines into three groups:

1. *Antipathic:* medicines that cause effects which are opposite to those of the disease.
2. *Homoeopathic:* medicines that cause effects similar to those of the disease.
3. *Allopathic:* medicines that cause effects that are neither similar nor opposite to those of the disease.

Self-healing Power of the Body

Symptoms such as sore throat or vomiting are seen as a sign that the body's self-healing powers are fighting infection. Homoeopathic medicines are designed not to suppress symptoms but to boost the body's vital force, or self-healing ability.

Suppression

In conventional medicine, the symptoms are considered to be a manifestation of the disease. The drugs are given to kill the bacteria causing it, or to dampen the symptom of the condition. Homoeopaths, on the other hand, see the symptoms as the body's attempt to heal itself. They see the symptom as a positive sign that the body's defence mechanism is trying to fight the underlying cause, and by this reasoning they insist that the symptoms should not be suppressed, as we are working against the body's attempt to cure it.

The initial meaning of suppression consisted of the belief that there are diseases whose external manifestations prevent development of inner symptoms of the same disease. In his *Chronic Diseases,* Hahnemann argued that mistreatment of diseases of the skin leads to disease deeper in the organism, listing numerous cases in support. Present day homoeopaths invoke this notion in claim that symptoms are not in themselves the disease, but rather represent an underlying disturbance of the organism's vitality. As they seek to address this underlying disease, homoeopaths do not automatically regard the disappearance of a symptom (whether spontaneous or in response to some treatment) as a favourable event. Under some cases this could instead indicate a weakening of the organism's ability to express the symptom, and because the underlying disturbance is still present, sooner or later it is expressed as a symptom elsewhere in the organism.

Homoeopaths further claim that the tendency of the past skin manifestations to reappear transiently following successful homoeopathic prescribing is considered an evidence in support of this notion. It is maintained that although suppression is sometimes necessary for the patient's welfare or may even be life-saving, it is regarded unfavourably in the context of long-term prognosis. In the modern context, the issue arises mainly with respect to the use of corticosteroid treatment for skin disease, allergies and asthma, and the use of chemotherapy, as homoeopathic treatment is claimed to be significantly less effective under immune-system suppression.

Aggravation

The phenomenon of existing symptoms worsening in response to homoeopathic treatment is termed as *homoeopathic aggravation.* Hahnemann refers to it as a healing crisis. The idea of aggravation can be considered a consequence of the law to be considered a consequence of the law of similars, whereby a remedy acts by accentuating the disease symptoms, thus promoting the organism's healing response. Some homoeopaths regard a quick aggravation as an indication of strong vitality, and tend to be encouraged by its presence, while others strive to avoid aggravations in favour of the patient's comfort throughout the treatment.

Potentiation

Another principle propagated by Hahnemann is the potentiation of the remedy. Homoeopathic medicines are diluted in alcohol or milk-sugar (lactose) or water to make them more palatable and also to reduce the harmful effects. It has been found that the more the medicine is diluted, the more effective and powerful it becomes. So, the process of the dilution is called potentiation, and the medicines are referred to as potencies. The crude homoeopathic medicine (example: cinchona) is triturated in alcohol to yield the mother tincture.

Individualisation

Treat the patient, not the disease – this is the most important doctrine of homoeopathy. No two human beings are alike, and so the medicines used for their treatment need not be alike. Homoeopathic medicines are prescribed based on the totality of symptoms of that individual. So, the name of the disease is not important to the doctor who tries to get a complete picture of the patient – his symptoms, the modalities of symptoms, his likes and dislikes, his environment, etc., to arrive at the individualised remedy. It is apt to sum up this in Charaka's words (*Samhita*):

"That alone is right medicine which can remove disease
He alone is the true physician who can restore health."

6

Case-taking

Homoeopathic remedies can be helpful in complex or even serious conditions, although self-prescribing is not appropriate in such cases. To correctly select the remedy and monitor the healing process, an experienced physician, who is trained in homoeopathy, should be involved, for the following reasons:-

1. Medical knowledge is needed to assess complex or serious conditions. Professional diagnostic tests may be necessary as well.
2. Using a remedy that covers isolated symptoms superficially, but does not fit the person on deeper levels, may change or suppress the symptoms, yet not be deeply curative.
3. Even with a correctly-chosen remedy, a temporary aggravation of symptoms may occur as part of the healing process. Training and experience are required to distinguish a helpful aggravation from an intensification of symptoms that occurs because a remedy has not acted and the illness is progressing.
4. An inexperienced or impatient person might be tempted to repeat the remedy unnecessarily, or change to other remedies at times when waiting is appropriate.

If an illness or condition is chronic or deep-seated, it is best to consult an experienced homoeopathic practitioner, for a 'constitutional' remedy that fits the characteristic symptoms of the case, and considers the person's physical condition and individual nature in a more comprehensive way. At a typical first visit, a homoeopath interviews a patient for at least an hour – to take a careful history and elicit information about many aspects of the person's state of health – before choosing a remedy.

The homoeopathic diagnostic method centres around what is called a case-taking of the patient's background, family conditions, hereditary body conditions, work situation, social situation, plus all the symptoms perceived by the patients and, preferably, also by persons close to the patient. By 'symptom' homoeopathic practice refers to anything perceived as not usual.

A homoeopath studies the whole person. Characteristics such as his temperament, personality, emotional and physical responses, when prescribing a remedy, are studied. So, a homoeopath may treat different persons exhibiting the same symptom differently. For example, two persons exhibiting flu-like symptoms may get two different medications from the homoeopath, based on the appraisal of the mind-body constitution.

A homoeopath would not prescribe one remedy for a person's headache, another for his stomach, and another for his depression. He tries to find a single remedy that creates the totality of symptoms that the person experiences. Homoeopathy is time-consuming for the practitioner and the patient, but is very effective in cure.

The first visit of a patient is important for the practitioner for which he needs to make certain preparations. The room where he will interview the patient should be well-lighted, comfortable and quiet.

When the patient is seated, the practitioner explains briefly the principles of homoeopathy so that the patient knows what to expect. Then he notes down his address, phone number, age, occupation, followed by the reason for his visit. The person is allowed to talk without interruptions about the nature of his illness. In homoeopathy, listening is crucial.

Through case-taking, the homoeopath gets to know many aspects of the patient, like restlessness, anxiety, skin colouring, eye contact, shyness, ease of communication. These observable symptoms are objective and valuable. He gathers information objectively and with compassion and patience.

After listening to the complaints, the homoeopath continues to ask general open questions about any additional symptoms until the interview is over.

For each symptom described, he will address the following:

1. When did you first have these symptoms? How old were you?
2. Have the symptoms changed over the years? How?
3. How often do these symptoms recur?
4. How long do these symptoms last?
5. Do you feel any sensations?
6. Does anything make it feel better?
7. Do you have any other symptoms accompanying your ailment?

A homoeopath must focus on etiology where the person's family history is included – all illnesses and predisposition, such as cancer, tuberculosis, HIV, emotional imbalances, diabetes, organ problems, and so on. He will also probe into the patient's past.

The following sample questions cover physical disharmonies, an important aspect of case-taking.

Appetite: Is it good or bad, explaining why?

Thirst: Do you feel very thirsty? How often do you drink, and how many glasses?

Food: What foods do you like or dislike? Any aversions? Does anything disagree?

Digestion: Do you have good bowel movements? Do you have any gas problem?

Urine: Any odour, unusual frequency? Do you wake up often at night to urinate? Unusual colour or blood?

Perspiration: Head or foot sweats? Sweaty palms? Unusual odour or excessiveness? Night sweats?

Skin: Dry, oily, acne, eczema, freckles, itches?

Energy: Is it normal, high or low? At what time of the day do you particularly feel so?

Sleep: Do you sleep well? If not, why? Is your sleep interrupted easily? Hard to go to sleep? Restless? The position you first take upon going to sleep? Do you feel refreshed on waking?

Dreams: Recurring or remembered? Feelings upon waking? Do you remember the dream?

Menses: Any headache, cramps, pains, nausea, irritability, cravings, unusual tendencies or related symptoms?

Sex: Desires high or low? Fantasies? Masturbation? Frequency of sexual release?

Body temperature: Usually more chilly or warm?

Seasons: Any preference? Why? Do you feel better or worse in a particular season?

Allergies: To what? What effects or symptoms?

Exercise: Do you like doing or not? How do you feel later?

Others: Anything else that you wish to add to your physical condition?

These simple questions make the patient feel safe enough to be honest and open about his emotions. With these preliminary questions, the homoeopath proceeds to question the patient about his mental make-up. The mental area is considered to be the most important aspect of case-taking in homoeopathy, because the practitioner gets an insight into the patient's psyche.

Questions relating to emotion and emotional tendencies are frequently difficult for both parties. But they need to be asked to fully understand the specific reactions of the patient. While emotions relate to feelings and energy, mental disturbances describe thought processes. They are given greater attention than physical symptoms. When emotions (energy in motion) are blocked, that says a great deal about the patient's behaviour.

There are specific questions addressed to the patient to get a clear picture of his core emotions. Each mental aspect or emotion is unique and important. They may be tedious at times, but should not be ignored.

Anger: How do you express your anger? Is it frequent? At whom is it expressed? How long do you remain angry? Any specific cases? Do you yell, scream, throw things or get violent?

Anxiety: Do you worry? About what specifically? Do you often worry? About the future, others, your health, money? Where in the body is it felt?

Company: Do you like to be alone or with people? Is solitude important?

Consolation: Do you like to be consoled or left alone? How do you feel while being consoled?

Sympathy: Are you sympathetic? Do you take up causes? How do you feel about animals.

Concentration: Do you find it difficult to concentrate? Do you experience any apathy? Confusion? Trouble with works or mistakes in speaking? Are you forgetful? Are you able to focus?

Critical: What are you critical about? In what manner? Are you judgemental about self! About other? How do you express it? Do you give in to sarcasm?

Depression: Do you ever feel depressed? How long does it last? What causes it? How is it shown? Any related physical symptoms? Any suicidal tendencies? Any intent or past attempts?

Excitable: How do you respond to a stimulus? Frequency? What is the common cause for it?

Fears: Have you had any fears in your childhood? Do you still have them? Any other fear?

Grief: Are you grieving over the loss of a loved one or a pet? How long has it lasted? Does any reference to it kindle feelings of grief? How recent has it been?

Impatience: What is the cause for it? Are you, by nature, impatient? How frequently do you become impatient in a day? Give examples.

Irritability: Cause and frequency? How long does it last? Is it related to food or allergy? Does loss of sleep make you irritable?

Jealousy: What triggers it and how frequently? Envy? Are you always suspicious by nature? Distrustful?

Guilt: About what? For how long?

Moods: High or low? Changing moods frequently or do you have stable moods? Any known causes?

Order: Are you fixated upon orderliness? Describe your office or your house and how orderly you like them to be. How organised or careless? Do you save things? Do you misplace them?

Reproach: Do you always like to blame others or find ways to justify your actions? Do you ever blame yourself? How is it expressed or felt? Do you scream or become violent?

Restlessness: Can you relax? Do you have the tendency to be always moving and be active? Do you have restless hands and feet?

Sensitivity: To what specifically? Are you sensitive to noises, odours, lights, emotions of others?

Weeping: Do you often cry? At what and how easily? Do you cry in privacy or even in the presence of others? While telling your symptoms do you cry? Do tears well up in your eyes when you are very angry?

Yielding: Do you try to avoid conflicts or do you like to air your grievance and settle the matter? Are you aggressive or submissive?

A practitioner will never ask leading questions, but try to make the patient talk as much as possible. During follow-up visits, patients report how they are responding to the remedy, which helps the practitioner make decisions about further treatment.

By looking at the whole person, certain symptoms become more prominent, along with the lifelong tendencies. After completing the case-taking, symptoms are analysed, reviewed and repertorised. Finally, the *Materia Medica* is researched to determine which remedy is most suitable for the patient.

7

The Importance of Repertory

A *repertory* is an index of symptoms, analysed and taken from provings, clinical experiences and self-experimentation. The symptoms are called *rubrics,* with related and corresponding remedies methodically arranged for ease.

Repertory originated from the Latin inventory. It is a table or a compendium where the contents are so arranged that they are easy to find. In homoeopathy, a repertory is an index of symptoms in *Materia Medica* with their corresponding homoeopathic medicines arranged systematically. It serves as a reference book and a guide for looking up a particular symptom or symptoms that may indicate the *similimum*. It helps homoeopaths to find the remedy, thus simplifying the work of selection of the most similar remedy.

The practice of homoeopathy started gaining popularity in Europe, USA and Asia. With new remedies being proved even after Hahnemann's death in 1843, the homoeopathic *Materia Medica* started to become voluminous. There was a need therefore to create an index of symptoms which would serve as easy reference for physicians. Hence, repertory gained importance.

Dr James Tyler Kent compiled one of the most comprehensive repertories available to the homoeopathic profession. It is the most popular and complete repertory. The first edition of this was published in 1897 in America. It is a product of long repertories. A later publication, William Boericke's *Repertory*, contains reference to 1414 homoeopathic drugs while Kent's includes only 591 drugs.

Repertories list illnesses, symptoms, modalities, both general and specific. The remedies included are especially useful in first-aid situations sudden or acute illness, seasonal illness, allergies, etc.

Repertories are similar to therapeutic or health guides in self-help books. A listing of ailments or symptoms are called rubrics in homoeopathy. First, the homoeopath finds the most troublesome symptom he is working to improve, and finds it on the A to Z listing of ailments. From there he will see a breakdown of the symptoms that help him to fine-tune his choice of remedy. For example, under 'Earache' he will see a further breakdown of symptoms that are all under the heading 'Earache'.

Earache

- First signs
- with redness and burning sensations
- painful
- inflammation
- middle ear
- in children
- right-sided

Next to each subheading is a remedy that matches.
A few examples are given below:

Abscesses

- red with swelling: *Belladonna 30C*
- helps pull out poisons: *Hepar Sulphur 30C*
- bluish: *Lachesis 30C*
- dental: *Mercurius Virus 30C*
- worse with cold: *Silicex 30C*

Abdominal Pain

- with gas: *Carbo Veg 30C*
- with spasmodic cramps: *Magnesium Phos 6X*

Acne

- *Juglans Reg 30C*

– worse with washing: *Sulphur 30C*

– teen acne: *Hepar Sulphur 30C*

It is well to remember one point in looking for symptoms in the repertory, and that is, when a practitioner cannot find the symptoms as given in the language of the patient, he should not despair, but look for some synonym until he finds what he is looking for. When he has found this, he should make a cross reference in his repertory so it will be easier the next time. Again, many fail to use the repertory because they think of symptoms in pathological terms. Symptoms are recorded in the *Materia Medica* in the language of the provers who were mostly laymen, and as the repertory is simply an index to the *Materia Medica,* the rubrics must be in their simple language.

Kent's version of the repertory is written in way unique to his thinking, his times and his homoeopathic experience. His first chapter, dealing with mental and emotional symptoms, starts with the word 'Abandoned' to the last rubric titled 'Wrong, everything seems'. His last chapter is 'Generalities'. One chapter focuses on the mind, after which are the following sections, each of which deals with physical disharmonies, and particular aspects of headings represent specific symptoms relating to those headings. His repertory, divided into the following 37 sections, are found in the order given below:

Mind, 1

Vertigo, 96 (time of day, when, where and physical sensations)

Head, 107 (including hair, headaches, pains, sensations and injuries)

Eye, 239 (sensations, discharges, eruptions, irritations and pain)

Vision, 275 (blurred, astigmatisms, colours, effected by, loss of)

Ear, 290 (abscess, discharge, eruptions, itch, noises, pain and wax)

Hearing, 326 (loss of, impaired and illusions)

Nose, 329 (*hay fever*, discharges, types of discharges, dryness, nosebleeds, fullness, itching, obstruction, pain and smell)

Coryza, 330

Epistaxis, 340

Discharges, 334

Smell, 354

Face, 360 (discolouration, expressions, eruptions, pain, heat and cold, wrinkles, ulcers, veins and swelling)

Mouth, 401 (abscesses, bleeding, discolouration, dryness, herpes, inflammation, odour, pain, tongue, salivation, speech, taste, swelling and tumours)

Tongue (found in many particulars)

Gums (also in many particulars)

Taste, 426

Speech, 423

Teeth, 435 (decay, discolouration, pain, looseness, grinding and sensitivity)

Throat, 452 (choking, discolouration, dryness, enlargement, heat, inflammation, irritation, mucus, pain, swallowing, sensitive, tonsils, spasms and ulcers).

External throat, 471 (glands, pain, goitre, stiffness, sensitivity and swellings)

Stomach, 478 (anxiety, appetite, food desires and aversions, constrictions, bloating, eructations, heartburn, heat, indigestion, nausea, pains, thirst and vomiting)

General symptoms referred through stomach are found under:

Appetite, 478

Aversion, 482

Desires, 485

Thirst, 529

The particulars are as:

Nausea, 506

Eructations, 491

Vomiting, 532

Continuing with the other sections.

Abdomen, 542 (anxiety, liver, distention, flatus, spleen, hernia, pains, inflammation, tension and ulcers)

Rectum, 605 (constipation, diarrhoea, haemorrhoids, bleeding, itch, pains, incontinence, prolapse, straining)

Constipation, 605

Diarrhoea, 608

Sleep, 1200 (disturbed, dreams, position, restless, insomnia, yawn, refreshing)

Chill, 1124 (time of day/year, sensations, exposure, internal, shivers, sides of the body)

Fever, 1242 (sensations, time, alternating, cerebro-spinal, cough, dry, continuous, perspiration, intensity, rash, gastric, intermittent, septic, sun, zymotic)

Perspiration, 1257 (time, causes, anxiety, exertion, odour, profuse sleep, suppressed)

Skin, 1267 (burning, itching, eruptions, herpes, shingles, hot/cold, discolouration, bruises, gangrene, freckles, inflammation, sensitive, sore, bites/stings, birthmarks, ulcers, warts, wrinkles)

Generalities, 1364 (aggravations covering the whole body, including time of day/year, anaemia, air, cancer, food, clothing, convulsions, lack of vital heat, faintness, injuries, loss of fluids, lassitude and weakness, motion, obesity, pains, pulse, sensitiveness, standing/sitting, swelling, touch, varicose veins, VD, wounds, and winds).

Many of our chronic cases may be worked out from these sections—mental and general.

Repertory Analysis, Dosage and Repetition

After the most difficult part of the task—that of individualising the patient's symptoms—has been completed, the selection of the remedy with the repertory is quickly done. Like all mathematical problems, the homoeopath starts with the right premises and follows certain axioms in order to arrive at the correct solution. Thus, if the logic of the symptom analysis is correct, if the technique of selection is without a flaw, the choice of the remedy must be mathematically certain.

One of the most difficult things to comprehend is when to repeat the dose. You will find as a general thing in acute cases that if a slight aggravation of the symptoms comes in a short time, you will not think of giving another dose, for the patient will get along better without more medicine, but there are conditions when it is necessary to repeat the dose. There is no clear-cut rule that can be laid down for this. Experience and powers of observation are essential for this. The basic and safe rule therefore is, never repeat the dose after reaction begins.

If more than one dose is necessary repeat the dose until there is improvement, and then stop; more doses will only retard the cure. When reaction is taking place never repeat the remedy; when reaction ceases or improvement stops, the remedy may be repeated.

Many good homoeopathic prescriptions are spoiled by too often repeated doses of the right remedy. We are often treating the effects of too many doses of the remedy when we think we are treating the disease. When the dilution of the right remedy carries the patient's case part way to health, and the practitioner is sure that he has the right remedy, he increases the strength of the remedy rather than changing to another unsuitable one. In this way he finds his cases being carried on to a complete cure. In *Chronic Diseases,* Hahnemann states,

> "The third leading mistake that the homoeopathic physician cannot too carefully or steadfastly avoid is in hastily and thoughtlessly giving some other medicine... but if once a medicine... is acting well and usefully, which is seen by the eighth or tenth day, then an hour or even half a day may come when a modern homoeopathic aggravation takes place. The good results may not appear in their best light before the twenty-fourth or thirtieth day. The dose will probably have then exhausted its favourable action about the fortieth or fiftieth day, and before that time it would be injudicious and an obstruction to the progress of the cure to give any other medicine. Experience teaches that a cure cannot be accomplished more quickly and surely than by allowing the suitable antipsoric to continue its action so long as improvement continues... Whoever can restrain his impatience as to this point will reach his object the more surely and the more certainly... periods of aggravation will occur, but so long as only the original ailments are renewed and no new, severe symptoms present themselves, they show a continuing improvement, being homoeopathic aggravations which do not hinder but advance the cure. The physician must, therefore, in chronic diseases, let all antipsoric remedies to act thirty, forty or even fifty and more days by themselves, so long as they continue to improve the

diseased state perceptibly to the acute observer; effects continue with the indicated doses, and these must not be disturbed and checked by new remedy."

When the homoeopath has given his remedy on the above formula, he may expect certain things to happen. In all curable cases he will expect a cure to take place or at least to be started. He may think that this cure is taking place by certain signs of nature which are given to him in the symptoms of the patient, and the way these signs or symptoms disappear will tell him if he is going to make a cure. If he is to cure, the symptoms must disappear from above downward, from within outward and in the reverse order in which they came.

Steps to Repertorisation

Repertorisation is not only a mechanical process of counting rubrics, it also includes the steps to reach the repertory proper, and finally differentiating the remedies with the help of *Materia Medica*. Repertory follows the logic of induction and deduction. The steps to repertorisation start from case-taking and end by finding out *similimum*. They are:

1. Case-taking
2. Recording and interpretation
3. Defining the problem
4. Classifications and evaluation of symptoms
5. Erecting totality
6. Selection of repertory and repertorisation
7. Repertorical result
8. Analysis and prescription

1. Case-taking

A case comprises symptoms which give the totality of a person's suffering. The totality of symptoms forms a case for the physician. In every event there exists a totality, provided an expert can perceive it. Likewise, in every alteration of state of health a totality exists which can be perceived by a physician.

Case-taking is the first step, and the outcome of treatment entirely depends upon the success of this first step. Any mistake committed here would certainly interfere in the selection of drugs and planning of the treatment.

Throughout the process of case-taking, the patient should be cooperative. He should be assured of the confidentiality of data. If he narrates well and fully, the task becomes easier for him and the physician. It should be a free exchange between them. Both verbal and non-verbal communication of the physician can either encourage or discourage the patient in opening up various events and their effects on him. To understand the feelings properly the physician should be an expert in role playing. He should acknowledge the feelings of the patient, but empathy should replace sympathy while dealing with sensitive cases.

At the end of the interview with the patient, the physician should have a clear definition of the problem. This is not always easy to achieve. If he remains in confusion at the level of case-taking, further steps in repertorisation would become intractable.

2. Recording and Interpretation

The need of a case record has been emphasised by all great practitioners for various essential purposes. Every case should be a piece of learning. Therefore, it is imperative to have it recorded clearly, so that the exact picture of the patient emerges. Very often it is noticed that all the information of the sick person do not find a place in case record, in which case the physician might unduly focus on some other effects which should be recorded without any interpolation or deletions.

Very often the use of technical terms can create confusion, so that should be avoided. Whatever the patient is trying to communicate should be properly received and interpreted by the physician, without any of his own prejudices creeping in.

The intensity of the symptoms should also be given due consideration while recording.

3. Defining the Problem

Once the case is recorded well, interpreted and analysed, the physician should be in a position to define the problem precisely. The record should give him to understand the person and his disease. The sickness of the person gets expressed at his various levels, and to bring all such expressions together to get a whole picture requires a clear understanding of what Hahnemann stated: "what is to be cured in a disease, that is to say, in every individual case of disease." To define a problem means to define the individual who is facing the problem. The diagnosis of the disease, which is of crucial importance, would segregate the peculiar characteristic expressions from the common ones. Thus, only by precisely defining the problem, a physician would be in a position to go ahead in the right direction.

4. Classification and Evaluation of Symptoms

It is a well-known fact that all the symptoms in a case are not equally important. After taking the case, a physician faces quite a big number of symptoms which are required to be analysed, classified and evaluated in order to arrange such symptoms hierarchically. Analysis and classification give an idea about the case in respect of its nature and the types of symptoms and, therefore, evaluation can be done by different methods.

According to Kent, the scheme of the order of importance of symptoms is:

a. *Mental:* will (emotion), understanding, intellect
b. *Physical:* time, temperature, weather, position, motion, external stimuli, eating, drinking, sleep, clothing and bathing.
c. *Particulars:* strange, rare and peculiar, and particular modalities.

All the three evaluation methods are to help the physician, and not to confuse him. After the case is well taken, evaluation of symptoms, according to the case, would not be difficult. The case may have different dimensions, which may prove useful to find out the *similimum.*

5. Erecting Totality

Totality is not the sum total of symptoms, but it is a logical combination of the symptoms which characterise the person as well as individualise the problem. Thus, all the symptoms which are classified and evaluated do not form a working totality of the case.

From the classification and evaluation, the hierarchy of symptoms is known, but which, among them, should be useful for getting a correspondence are yet to be finalised. Thus, a physician is required to understand all the symptoms and select a few of which can logically represent the whole picture. This logical arrangement must follow a definite principle. If the case has got more generals and a few particulars with rare modalities, it would follow a different arrangement than a case which has vague modalities and striking concomitants, or a pathological general.

Totality should be erected according to the facts collected in the case. There is no hard and fast rule to erect totality in any fixed way. The case alone decides the method to be followed.

6. Selection of Repertory and Repertorisation

After the totality has been erected, the case becomes clear to the physician. He should look for one of the following points in the case:

    a. *Generals*: mentals, physicals

    b. *Particulars*: location, sensation, modalities, concomitants

    c. *Pathological generals*

Once the repertory is selected, a major part of the analysis and synthesis of the case is done. The next step is to rearrange the totality according to the repertory selected. Rearrangement of the totality in terms of repertory selected is called *Repertorial Totality*. Thus, a well-arranged totality is worked out.

What follows next is to convert the symptoms into rubrics which requires an acquaintance with the repertory. The symptoms obtained from the patient may not be found in the repertory in the same form. So the physician must know the construction and arrangement of each repertory. Rubrics should be arranged according to hierarchy, reason and page number.

7. Analysis and Prescription

Repertorial result should be referred to the *Materia Medica*. Further, the group has to be referred to the picture of the patient and with the help of the *Materia Medica,* it should be differentiated.

Repertory thus narrows down the group of medicines and with the help of source books, a final remedy can be found out. The remedy so selected must finally pass through certain criteria such as susceptibility, sensibility, suppression (if any), the level of similarity, functional and structural changes, vitality and miasm, to arrive at the right potency and the schedule of the doses .

8

Materia Medica

The *Materia Medica* is a dictionary of homoeopathic medicines and their symptoms. It is a book which is the final authority on homoeopathy. It contains the properties of medicines, properties which have been proved on healthy individuals.

Homoeopathic doctors rely on the *Materia Medica* as the authority, for it contains not empty theories, but details of symptoms which were experienced by hundreds of provers. It is thus a system based on sound principles and as a result of solid experiments.

The symptoms are arranged in a systematic order—Mind Head, Eyes, etc. It is not required for a doctor to memorise or remember all the contents of the *Materia Medica*. What is required is to understand the nature or keynotes of each remedy.

A number of provings were compiled by Hahnemann into this great work called *Materia Medica,* and this was later expanded by his followers. The idea of homoeopathic treatment is that the patient's symptom profile is taken, then the *Materia Medica* is carefully perused to find the medicine that provides the best (ideally perfect) match of that symptom profile. That is assumed to be the medicine which cures that particular case. During this matching, interestingly, a medicine is sought that matches as many of the patient's symptoms as possible, whereas any symptom recorded for the medicine, but not matching the patient's profile, are normally ignored. According to Hahnemann, some unspecified selective mechanism ensures that the right properties of the medicine are activated. This is very practical since most medicines have many symptoms on their list, sometimes hundreds.

As Clarke says, "There is no road to the practice of homoeopathy (whether it is the clinical road or the symptomatic road) which does not entail close and constant study of *Materia Medica.*" And as Kent says, "The artistic prescriber must study the *Materia Medica* long and earnestly to enable him to fix in his mind sick images." Therefore, constant study of the *Materia Medica* and constant use of the repertory are essential since we have to acquaint ourselves with the repertorial rubrics.

There is no doubt that the *Materia Medica* of Hahnemann is an enduring monument to the genius of its author, original in its conception and design, and unique in its form and contents. Its foundation is on the bedrock of natural law. Over its portals are etched the words, *Similia, Similibus, Curantur; Simplex, Similimum, Minimum.*

The task of mastering the *Materia Medica,* vast and even impossible as it seems, is comparatively simple. The needle that points the way through the seeming wilderness of the symptoms is the principle of *Similia* —the remedial law of homoeopathy. The reason for the existence of this precious look in its characteristic form becomes evident when the drug symptoms recorded in it are seen to be exact counterparts of the symptoms of the disease, and it is explained that medicines cure disease by virtue of this similarity of symptoms. The arrangement of symptoms according to an anatomical scheme is for the purpose of comparison—symptoms of drugs with the symptoms of disease.

A number of *Materia Medicas* have been authored. Prominent among them are listed below:

Kent's Lectures on Homoeopathic Materia Medica: This is an excellent source for 180 remedies, giving a detailed approach to Kent's unique work.

Boericke's Materia Medica with Repertory: Included in this book are a vast majority of remedies, somewhat outdated in its terminology, but there are also included less detailed remedies.

J H Clark's Dictionary of Materia Medica: This book has practically all remedies, with specific characteristics.

Gibson's Studies of Homoeopathic Remedies: This book includes 120 remedies with sources, clinical notes and general appearance.

Hering's Condensed Materia Medica: A single volume condensed from ten volumes.

Morrison's Desktop Guide: This covers 200 remedies, with updated terminology, clinical aspects and comparisons.

Murphy's Lotus Materia Medica: A modern, insightful book with 1,200 remedies, incorporating remedy folklore.

The symptoms, experienced by the provers, are written in plain and common terms in these books. Instead of the technical language of the medical profession, the one used here is the language of everyday use. The *Materia Medica* is not subject to the influence of the transitory theories of general medicine, with its constantly changing terminology and bewildering array of newly invented terms.

Morrison's Desktop Guide covers 156 polycrests (or remedies) in detail, providing an overall picture for each.

Please remember that the following list is for general information only. Homoeopathic medicine should be selected considering totality of symptoms. For selection of correct medicine, dose and potency, you should consult your homoeopath.

Aconitum Napellus (Acon)
Sudden appearance of complaints; extreme restlessness; great fears (specially of death); anxiety; influenza; dryness of mouth, throat and skin with intense thirst for cold water; anxious dreams.

Aesculus Hippocastanum (Aesc)
Dry and swollen mucous membranes; haemorrhoids; burning of anus after stool; backache.

Aethusa Cynapium (Aeth)
Intolerance of milk; stool undigested, thin, greenish, preceded by colic.

Allium Cepa (All-c, also Cepa)
Watery and acrid nasal discharge which becomes worse in warm room; oppressed breathing; tickling in larynx; eyes become sensitive to light.

Aloes (Alo)
Sense of insecurity in rectum; stool passes without effort; taste becomes bitter; diarrhoea from beer.

Alumina (Alum)
Very severe constipation; no desire for days: rectum sore and dry; dryness of mucous membranes.

Anacardium (Anac)
Low self-esteem; abusive; cursing; depression; fears and delusions; controlling, violent and angry; brain fatigue, most symptoms better from eating; strong sexual desires.

Antimonium Crudum (Ant-C)
Excessive irritability; tongue thickly-coated white; loss of appetite; menses suppressed from cold bathing, watery leucorrhoea; various skin diseases; arthritic pain in fingers.

Antimonium Tartaricum (Ant-t)
Respiratory problems; rattling of mucous but little expectoration; thirst for cold water but little and often; great drowsiness.

Apis Mellifica (Apis)
Oedema of skin and mucous membranes; stinging pains; intolerance of heat; no thirst; swelling in the throat; swelling after insect bites; last drops of urine burn and smart; inflammation of kidneys.

Argentum Nitricum (Arg-n)
Patient is always in hurry; headache from mental exertion; symptoms of in-coordination; painful swelling of the pit of stomach; great desire for sweets; intolerance of heat; sexual weakness in males; diarrhoea immediately after eating or drinking.

Arnica Montana (Arn)
Traumatic injuries; pain from overuse of an organ; fetid breath; violent spasmodic cough; angina pectoris; small boils; thrombosis; tinnitus.

Arsenicum Album (Ars)
Influenza with thin; watery and excoriating nasal discharge; Sneezing; photophobia; seaside complaints; restlessness; food poisoning; intolerance of smell of food; jaundice; anaemia; skin – dry; rough; scaly; psoriasis which is worse in winters; periodic fever; typhoid; thoughts of committing suicide.

Aurum (Aur)
Severe suicidal depression; serious; self-condemnation; guilt and abandonment issues; worse during cloudy weather; worse with pain; anger with remorse; moans during sleep.

Baptisia (Bapt)
Septic conditions; fetid breath; stool offensive thin, dark, bloody; menses too early, too profuse; sleeplessness and restlessness; nightmares and frightful dreams.

Baryta Carbonica (Bar-C)
Tonsils; and glands around ears painful and swollen; easy taking of cold; abdomen hard and tense; palpitation when lying on left side; fetid foot sweat.

Belladonna (Bell)
Sudden and violent complaints and inflammations; neuralgic pains which come and go suddenly; no thirst; redness of affected organs; skin sore and sensitive; dysmenorrhoea; menses profuse; eyelids red and swollen; epistaxis; spasmodic hiccough.

Berberis Vulgaris (Berb-V)
Kidney and gall bladder stones; inflammation of kidneys; bloody urine; anal fistula; itching of skin worsened by scratching; lumbago.

Bryonia Alba (Bry)
Excessive irritability; dryness of all mucous membranes; great thirst for large quantities of water; constipation; menses suppressed; frequent bleeding of nose when menses should appear; dry cough; joints red and swollen; all complaints are aggravated by motion.

Calcarea Carbonicum (Calc-C or Calc)
Apprehension; forgetfulness; excessive sweat of head; discharge from ears; easy taking of cold; head proportionately larger but legs

thinner in children; obesity; loss of appetite when tired; umbilical
hernia; gallstone colic; menses too early, too profuse and too long;
feet feel cold and damp.

Calcarea Phosphorica (*Calc-P*)
Complains constantly about everything; craves for smoked food;
feels weak; always dissatisfied; loves change and travel.

Cantharis (*Canth*)
Abdominal complaints which are aggravated by coffee;
inflammation of urinary passages; constant urge to urinate; nephritis
with bloody urine; excessive sexual desires in females; burns and
scalds; irregular pulse; pericarditis.

Carbo Vegetabilis (*Carb-V*)
Lowered vital power; deficiency of oxygen in the body; very slow;
hands and feet cold; epistaxes; distress even from simplest food;
flatulent colic; pulse imperceptible; easy fainting.

Carcinosin (*Carc*)
Intense, sympathetic, passionate; family history of cancer;
fastidious; craves chocolates and spicy food; moles on back; strong
libido; loves animals; low energy from 3 pm to 6 pm; loves travel.

Causticum (*Caust*)
Chronic rheumatic; arthritic and paralytic affectations; paralysis
of tone and vocal chords; unsteadiness of muscles; involuntary
passing of urine specially at night and in the aged.

Chamomilla (*Cham*)
Excessive irritability and impatience, especially in children; violent
earache; diarrhoea of children during dentition; tickling cough;
rheumatic pains.

Cina
Worm affectations; bed wetting; grinding of teeth; pale face with
dark rings around the eyes.

China officinalis (*Cinch or China*)
General weakness; aversion to mental or physical exertion; ringing
in ears; violent, dry sneezing; ill effects of tea; weakness due to
loss of fluids; painless frothy stools; slow digestion; distention of
stomach and abdomen after eating; hiccough; jaundice.

Colocynthis (Coloc)
Intense abdominal pain causing the patient to bend over double; dysentery; taste very bitter; contraction of muscles; stiffness of joints.

Conium (Con)
Emotional flatness or indifference; paralysis; cancer; hardness of glands; tumours; fixed ideas; fogginess of the brain.

Cuprum (Cupr)
Spasms and convulsions; appears emotionally closed; sensation as if suffocating; flat facial expression; seizures; rigid; intense emotions suppressed.

Drosera Rotundifolia (Dros)
Spasmodic, dry, irritating, choking cough (much like whooping-cough) with hoarseness of voice; nose bleed, disinclination to speak because talking creates breathing difficulties.

Eucalyptus Globulus (Cucal)
This is a powerful antiseptic; relapsing fever; slow digestion; dysentery; nephritis; high fever; asthma.

Euphrasia (Euphr)
Burning and swelling of eyelids; watering eyes with many other eye troubles; prostatitis.

Ferrum Metallicum
Anaemia; desires raw meat; overweight; face flushes easily; very sensitive to noise; strong-willed; better walking slowly; general weakness and fatigue; demanding.

Gelesemium (Gels)
Various degrees of motor paralysis; muscular weakness; vertigo; insomnia; dim-sightedness; diarrhoea from emotional excitement.

Graptutes (Graph)
Dryness of skin; nails deformed and brittle; constipation; obesity; hot drinks create problems; offensive breath.

Hamamelis Virginica (Ham)
Bleeding haemorrhoids; haemorrhage from any part; varicose veins; orchitis.

Hepar Sulphuris Calcareum (Hep)
Great sensitiveness to all impressions; tendency to suppuration; cough when exposed to dry and cold wind; chronic and recurring urticaria; deep cracks on hands and feet; great sensitiveness to dry; cold weather.

Hyoscyamus (Hyos)
Paranoia, jealous with violent outbursts; intense sexual desires; worse with touch; hyperactive child; shameless; defiant; delusions; talkative; fear of dogs; wild gestures.

Hypericum Perforatum (Hyper)
Relieves post-operative pains; useful for injuries to nerves; tetanus; crawling sensation in hands and feet.

Ignatia Amara (Ign)
Many of the emotional symptoms including ill effects of grief and worry; changeable moods; twitching of facial muscles; insomnia; violent yawning; dry spasmodic cough; feminine sexual frigidity; coffee aggravates many problems.

Iodum (Iod)
Very warm; thyroid dysfunctions; very restless and busy; compulsive; talkative and anxious; impulsive; intense appetite; anger; avoids company; discontent; and destructive; general fears.

Ipecacuanha (Ip or Ipec)
Nausea and vomiting due to any reason; haemorrhages where blood is bright red; diarrhoea with grass-green stool; profuse uterine haemorrhage; asthma; bleeding from lungs; sleep with eyes half open; suffocating and wheezing cough.

Kali Bichromicum (Kali-b)
Thick, ropy secretions; loss of smell; stomach ulcer; left-sided sciatica; quick migration of pains; cirrhosis of liver.

Kali Carbonicum (Kali-C)
Sharp and cutting pains; sensitiveness to weather changes; dryness and falling out of hair; sour eructations; weakness of back; large haemorrhoids; pulse weak, rapid and intermittent; cold weather complaints.

Kali Phosphoricum (Kali-P)

Weakness of nervous system; mental and physical depression; loss of memory; humming and buzzing in the ears; severe dysentery.

Kreosotum (Kreos)

Ulcerations; cancerous affectations; very painful dentition; rapid decay of teeth; hoarseness; cholera of infants; senile gangrene. cracking of soles.

Lachesis Mutus (Lach)

Climactic hot flushes; toothache; diphtheria; quinsy and many other complaints related with throat and respiratory system; neuralgia of coccyx.

Ledum Palustre (Led)

Rheumatism; goity nodosities; anal fissures; carbuncles; complaints which appear from below upwards.

Lycopodium (Lyc)

Lack of self-confidence; weakness of memory; night blindness; anorexia; small quantities of food create fullness; distention of abdomen; cirrhosis; hernia; painful haemorrhoids; sciatica; impotence; psoriasis; hepatitis.

Magnesia Muriatica (Mag-m)

Yielding; aversion to confrontations; feels anxious at night; very responsible; noises annoy; composed, with suppressed inner anger; depression; unrefreshing sleep.

Magnesia Phosphorica (Mag-p)

Spasmodic pains; cramps of muscles; toothache; flatulent colic; menstrual colic; angina pectoris; spasmodic palpitation.

Medorrhinum (Medo)

Nasal discharges; cruel and aggressive behaviour; an extremist; self-centred and loves danger; obsessive/compulsive; history of VD; hurried; intense passions; bites fingernails; overwhelmed by impulses; night person; loves sea.

Mercurius Solubilis (Merc)

Secondary stage of syphilis; profuse and burning discharge from eyes; yellow; bloody discharge from ears; sneezing in sunshine;

swelling of nasal bones; spongy and easily bleeding gums; intense thirst for cold drinks; paralysis of the aged.

Mercurius Sublimatus Corrosivus (Merc-C)
Gonorrhoea; inflammation and soreness of eyes; red, swollen and painful throat; bloody dysentery; sensitiveness of epigastrium.

Natrum Muriaticum (Nat-m)
Great weakness; high blood pressure and even low pressure; blinding headache; violent and fluent coryza, especially which begins with sneezing; numbness of tongue; tachycardia; pulse intermits on lying down; falling out of hair.

Natrum Carbonicum (Nat-C)
Very sensitive; craves potatoes; inner turmoil and depression with appearance of cheerfulness; prefers solitude; emotionally closed; sweet and selfless; delicate; poor digestion; worse in heat and sun; sadness; milk allergies; sympathetic.

Natrum Sulphuricum (Nat-S)
Head injuries and concussions; suicidal depression; very responsible and serious; warm blooded; feels better after a bowel movement; emotionally closed; asthma; possible past history of venereal disease; sensitive; practical, with business focus.

Nitricum Acidum (Nit-A)
Generally negative person; selfish; discontent; anger; curses; restless; hypersensitive; selfish; anxieties about health and death; vindictive; chilly; pains come and go suddenly.

Nux Vomica (Mux-v)
Great irritability; habit of finding faults with others; headache in sunshine and on waking in the morning; nose stuffed up at night; stomach problems are aggravated by eating; frequent ineffectual urging for stool; blind haemorrhoids; dysmenorrhoea; asthma due to digestive disorders; unrefreshing sleep.

Opium (Op)
Lack of response to various medicines; vertigo; fright; delirium; paralysis of tongue; obstinate constipation; stool round like black balls; snoring; great drowsiness; convulsions; useful in coma.

Petroleum (Petro)
Skin disharmonies of all types, with dryness; quick temper; motion sickness; herpes; offensive perspiration; unable to make decisions; chilly; worse in winter; increased hunger.

Phosphoricum Acidum (Phos A)
Dullness and slowness; apathy; feels overwhelmed with grief and emotions; intense fatigue and loss of energy; yielding; desires refreshing fruits; dehydration; chilly.

Phosphorus (Phos)
Great lowness of spirit; dread of death when alone; fatty degenerations; scurvy; vertigo of the aged; dandruff; falling of hair; haemorrhages; cirrhosis of liver; glaucoma; epistaxis instead of menses; vomiting soon after taking water; hoarseness; various respiratory problems.

Phytolacca Decandra (Phyt)
Loss of personal delicacy; indifference to life; dark redness of throat with swollen tonsils; quinsy; mumps; cancer and abscess of breast; urine suppressed with pain in kidney region.

Platinum
Primarily a female remedy; haughty to the extreme; is worse with touch; idealistic; dwells on the past; feels abandoned; dislikes children; insolent and rude; pretentious; strong libido.

Plumbum (Plum)
Taciturn; sad; shy; selfish; difficulty in expressing oneself; indifference; illness slow in development; very chilly; pains tend to radiate; neurological disorders.

Podophyllum (Pod)
Profuse, painless, watery, gushing diarrhoea; internal and external piles; grinding of teeth at night.

Psorinum (Psor)
Skin dysfunction of all types; periodicity; pessimist; tend to despair with hopelessness; anxiety and fear especially of poverty; very chilly; low energy; feels forsaken and lost; dirty skin.

Pulsatilla Nigra (Puls)

Patient is timid and can be easily discouraged; moods are changeable and contradictory; mouth is dry but no thirst; taste of mouth keeps changing; secretions from eyes; nose and mouth are sick, dislike for fatty and warm food; menses delayed, scanty, thick, dark, clotted, intermittent and changeable; pains in the body keep shifting; styes; acne; measles.

Rhus Toxicodendron (Rhus-t)

Extreme restlessness; thoughts of suicide; rheumatic pains which are worse at the beginning of motion; drowsiness after eating; pains due to over-exertion; pain and stiffness in small of back; sciatica; urticaria; complaints are worse when at rest.

Ruta

Affects tendons and fibrous tissues; startles easily; distrustful; argumentative; stiffness and pain; strains and sprains; eyestrain; related headaches; worse motion or lying on painful side.

Sepia (Sep)

Indifference to friends and relatives; chronic nasal catarrh; herpes behind ears; nausea in morning before eating; desire for spicy food; irregular menses with bearing down sensation; weakness of back; hot flushes at menopause.

Silica (Sil)

Intolerance of alcoholic stimulants; tendency to formation of pus; styes; boils and abscesses; constipation before and after menses; extreme coldness of body with desire to remain close to the fire; offensive foot sweat; crippled nails; keloid growths; loss of smell.

Spigelia (Spig)

Pericarditis violent palpitation; angina pectoris; rheumatic carditis and other problems related to the heart; left-sided headache.

Spongia (Spon)

Fear of suffocation; heart ailments; increased anxiety; dry mucus membranes; dry, barking croupy cough; easily frightened; thyroid disharmonies; respiratory conditions; weakness.

Staphysagria (*Staph*)

Sweet; yielding person; suppressed emotions; very sensitive; emotionally dependent; fear of losing control; possible history of sexual abuse or humiliation; strong sexual history; grief; suppressed anger; low self-confidence, worse after a nap.

Stramonium (*Stram*)

Violent tendencies; etiology from a fright; impulsive rage; wild behaviour; night terror; desires company and light; intense thirst; flushed face; excitable; stammers; convulsions; promiscuous; hyperactive children; could be mild, gentle and very sensitive.

Sulphur (*Sulph*)

Forgetfulness; burning and redness of eyes; burning in palms and soles; unhealthy skin with tendency to skin diseases; excess acidity; difficult respiration; aversion to bathing; haemorrhoids.

Syphilinum (*Syph*)

Compulsive tendencies, worse at night; very chilly; alcoholic; excess saliva; fear of disease or germs or going insane; nails are distorted; anxious; indifferent; worse hot or cold extremes.

Thuja Occidentalis (*Thuy*)

Fig-warts; freckles; fungus growths; loss of appetite; rapid emaciation; constipation with violent rectal pain; piles; gonorrhoea; asthma in children.

Tuberculinum (*Tuber*)

Desires change and travel; feels unfulfilled; can be mean; compulsive; chilly; respiratory disharmonies; milk and cat allergies; desires smoked food; hyperactive children; romantic longings; excess perspiration at night; itch; better with heat.

Veratrum Album (*Verat*)

Extreme coldness; blueness and weakness; pale face; painful diarrhoea followed by great weakness; weakness of heart with intermittent action; cramps in calves.

Zincum Metallicum (*Zinc*)

Sensitivity to noise; lethargy; headache due to wine or liquor; squinting of eyes; cholera of infants; weakness; trembling and twitching of various muscles of limbs; backache.

These remedies are only a select few that have been listed from 2,500 remedies available. Nevertheless, about 75 per cent of all cases can be well served by using one of the above polycrests. Remember, these are only for an understanding of how the system of homoeopathy functions.

The above remedies are the ones most frequently prescribed, and most often listed in repertories.

9

Potentiation

Another cornerstone of homoeopathy is the potentiation of medicines. Potentiation is a process that involves a series of precise dilutions and succussions (a vigorous shaking action). A substance has to undergo this process to be useful as a homeopathic remedy.

"Homoeopathic potentiation is a mathematico-mechanical process for the reduction, according to scale, of crude, inert or poisonous medical substances to a state of physical solubility, physiological assimilability and therapeutic activity and harmlessness, for use as homoeopathic healing remedies" (Stuart Close, *The Genius of Homoeopathy*).

The primary object of potentiation is to reduce all substances designed for therapeutic use to "a state of approximately perfect solution or complete ionisation, which is fully accomplished only by infinite dilution" (Arrhenius). The greater the dilution, the higher is the degree of ionisation, until, at infinite dilution, ionisation is complete and therapeutic activity conditionally greatest.

"To Hahnemann alone is due imperishable honour and renown for discovering, first the existence of a universal law of cure, and, second, that the specific properties of drugs could be developed, transmitted and utilised by potentiation," writes Morgan.

Some of the basic substances tried by Hahnemann were quite toxic, and caused some unpleasant, possibly even dangerous, poisoning effects. Obviously, apart from making testing dangerous, it would hardly seem expedient to add to the sufferings of sick people by giving them toxic substances, especially since that was exactly what Hahnemann was blaming other practitioners for. So Hahnemann started diluting his substances, using a special procedure of vigorous shaking which he called 'succussion'. For instance, he put a drop of raw substance into a vial, added 100 drops of dilution medium (water or alcohol), succussed it, then repeated the process several times. After n steps, the dilution, or potency, he called nC.

Potentiation is very important, because the repeated process of dilution and succussion brings about an energetic change that gives the substance a deeper curative effect. Repeated dilution removes all chances of chemical toxicity, allowing the homoeopathic use of many substances that would otherwise not be safe to take as a medicine.

Potentiation is also known as dynamisation. While liquids are diluted as they are with water or alcohol, insoluble solids are diluted by grinding them with lactose, a process known as trituration. Homoeopathic practitioners believe that the vigorous agitation following each dilution transfers some of the essential properties of the substance to the water, which fits in with the concept of the disease as a substance in the vital force of the patient.

The dilution factor at each stage is traditionally 1:10 (D or x potencies) or 1:100 (C potencies). Hahnemann advocated the use of 30C dilutions for most purposes, that is, dilution by a factor of 100^{30}–10^{60}. Critics point out that, since Avogadro's number is only 6.022×10^{23} particles, the chance that even one molecule of the original would be present in a 15C solution is small, and the chance of one molecule of the original present in a 30C solution is infinitesimal.

Some homoeopaths, in particular Kent, advocated the use of much higher potencies, whose manufacture could no longer be practically achieved by the traditional methods, but required succussion without dilution, higher dilution factors, or machines which in some way integrate dilution and succussion into a continuous process.

Higher dilutions are generally considered stronger and deep-acting. This is in contrast to pharmacology and biochemistry, which hold that the effects of a substance are always due to its physical or biochemical activity in the patient's body, and, therefore, that generally the more of an active ingredient is present in a drug, the more effect (whether positive, negative, or both) it will have. The choice of potency will depend on a number of factors. These include how deep-seated the disease appears to be, whether the disease is primarily physical or more mental/emotional, the patient's sensitivity based on the practitioner's intuitive assessment or previous reactions to remedies; and the desired dosing regimen based on patient compliance considerations (for example, low potency repeated vs high potency repeated seldom). There are many theories and traditions of use of potency. For example, as a general rule, French and German homoeopaths use lower potencies than their American counterparts. What most homoeopaths agree on is that the choice of potency is secondary to the choice of remedy. A well-chosen remedy will act in a variety of potencies, but an approximately matched remedy might act only in certain potencies.

It is widely accepted that the simplest part of homoeopathy to address scientifically is potentised medicines. Basically, preparations over 12C consist of shaken medium, and even lower potencies contain so little substance that it can hardly have any chemical effect. Homoeopathic proponents hold that the medium somehow conveys the effect of the original substance. There is no known mechanism within modern physics that can explain how this could happen, and no scientific disciplines within physics or chemistry have ever shown any effects that might hint at water (or alcohol) having any memory of substances no longer present.

Potency

1x potency of the medicine signifies 1 part of mother tincture diluted with 9 parts of alcohol/milk sugar.

2x potency is 1x of medicine diluted with 9 parts of sugar milk/alcohol.

1C potency is mother tincture diluted with 99 parts.

1 M potency is mother tincture diluted with 999 parts.

Low potency: 1x, 3x, 63 (3C), 12x(6C)

Medium potency: 12x, 30x, 30C

High potency: 200C, 1M, 20M, CM, LM, etc.

The potency of a remedy such as 6x or 30C says how many times and by what ratio the base substance has been diluted. The purpose of potency is to dilute the remedy until it can do no harm, and to potentise (or invigorate) the base substance with energy such that the qualities are preserved while the substance itself is diluted out. Tincture is where it begins. In most remedies, the tincture is made by steeping the powdered base substance in alcohol. Insolubles, like mercury, are made by thoroughly mixing the substance in powdered lactose.

What potency should you take? Just remember, higher is not always better. Hahnemann only used potencies under 30x, and his record is impressive. It is best to start at the lowest potency that fits the problem, especially if the symptoms are mostly physical.

The lower the potency, the more general the application. So if the homoeopath does not have the right remedy, he has a better chance of a response with lower than with high potencies. Low potencies can be repealed much more often, and are less likely to provoke strong healing aggravations. The higher the potency, the more precise the selection needs to be, and the deeper it can resonate, especially into the mental/emotional realm. It would be advisable that potencies above 200C should be the exclusive domain of licensed professionals and constitutional case work, as they should not be repeated often; their effects can be subtle and are not always measurable to the untrained eye.

Another general rule for potency is that the faster, more severe the onset of a problem, the higher the potency one can use. One can knock out a sudden, severe, very restless flu quite quickly with a few doses of a fast acting remedy like 30C *Nux* or *Belladonna* repeated every 15 minutes, whereas a slower moving flu like Bryonia's is generally better off with 6x-30x, taken three or four times a day as needed when symptoms flare up. A blow to the head obviously needs the highest *Arnica* on hand whereas a stubbed toe can be mended with a simple 6x dose. As Hering's Law states, "The faster the onset, the faster the exit."

Individual sensitivity is another factor in determining potency. If an individual is very sensitive to his surroundings, the environment, foods, smells or prior medications that have been taken, then they will also be sensitive to the remedies, LM or 6C to 12C potencies with infrequent repetition is best in such circumstances, especially when used in water solutions. The selection of the best potency is a matter of individual experience and observation, not a matter of laws.

To sum up in the words of Stuart Close, "In general, it may be stated that any curable disease may be cured by any potency, when the indicated remedy is administered; but that cure may be much accelerated by selecting the potency or dose appropriate to the individual case."

10

Miasms

The word 'miasm' is derived from the Greek word *miainein,* meaning 'to pollute or stain'. It denotes a cloud or fog in the being. Miasms are like echoes of the original physical illnesses or toxic poisons that are given to us by both our family lines or acquired during our lifetime. They are resonances of negativity or harmful vibrations powered from these original physical illnesses or poisonous substances. Unless they are eliminated, they last for our entire lives. They attract toxic poisons present in the bloodstream, and layer them into the connective tissue from where they set up a predisposition to illness in the lifetime of the person.

A miasm is an inherited genetic state given to you by both your family lines from which subsequent generations carry the negative resonance of the original poison or poisons.

Take, for instance, the case of a person getting chickenpox at a young age. The mother will cover the marks with calamine lotion or hydrocortisone cream, thus suppressing the symptoms of the disease—the symptoms that are so important for indicating that he is unwell. The suppression leads the disease inwards where it will reside in hiding (on the ends of the nerves in this case) as a miasm of the original chickenpox. Later in life that person will provably suffer a painful bout of shingles caused by the original virus being suppressed and not eliminated. If the shingles is also suppressed, there is herpes zoster miasm to the sixth generation where skin problems will be to the fore in each preceding generation. This is nature's way of finally trying to rid the body of the virus by forcing it out through the skin. As the bowel and lung are related to the skin, further generations will be prone to lung and bowel problems throughout their lives.

During the eighteenth century, the word 'miasm' was loosely used to denote the discharge coming from decaying animal or vegetable matter. It was also sometimes used to denote the discharge coming from the bodies of diseased persons. The agents, which were thought to be connected with the production of disease, were designated by a general term 'miasm' or 'miasma'.

The use of the term by Hahnemann remains controversial. At some places in his writing, Hahnemann has used *miasm* to denote the predisposition for disease, and at other places he has used it to denote the disease-causing agent, similar to bacteria and viruses, and the states arising from their suppression.

Hahnemann used the term 'miasm' to describe the trans-generational causes to disease. He asserted that unless this 'obstacle to cure' was dealt with, the cure of the disease would always be incomplete.

History of Miasms

Hippocrates was the first physician to use the term 'miasm' which has its origin in the Greek word for taint or fault. He postulated that certain infectious diseases were transmitted to humans by air and water tainted by miasms. In the late eighteenth century it was a common belief that miasms were impure airs that were responsible for the spread of epidemic diseases among groups of people. Hahnemann realised that the air could carry infectious diseases but he did not consider the pathogenic material to be gaseous in nature.

In the early days of his practice, when he started using the law of similars, he got good results in acute and epidemic diseases, but he failed miserably in a large number of chronic diseases. He himself said, "Their beginning was promising, the continuation less favourable, the outcome hopeless...." For example, if a patient came to him with pain in knee, worse by initial motion and better by continued motion, he would have probably prescribed *Rhus tox*. If the cause of this symptom was acute, the patient would get cured. If the case was chronic (say, gout or arthritis), the patient would often come back with the same symptoms after an initial amelioration.

Such instances made Hahnemann probe deeply into the concept of disease and the development of the chronic diseases. After 12 years of detailed case-takings and case analysis, he found out that nearly all the patients with chronic diseases had a history of either scabies, syphilis or gonorrhoea, and most of the patients were not well since the time of infection. He called these infections and the tendency arising from them, miasms. The one arising from scabies was called psora or non-venereal miasm. The other two were called venereal miasms as they arose from sexual conduct. The one arising from syphilis was called syphilitic miasm, and the one from gonorrhoea was called sycotic miasm.

These things Hahnemann wrote about in his theory of diseases. The theory of miasms originates in his book, *Chronic Diseases,* which was published in 1828, around the same time that he decided to fix 30C as the standard potency for all homoeopaths. He declared that the theory was the result of 12 years of the most painstaking work on difficult cases of a chronic character combined with his own historical research into the diseases of man.

Hahnemann states in *The Organon,* "The suffering of the immediate vital principle which animates the interior of our bodies, when it is morbidly disturbed, produces symptoms in the organism that are manifest. The physician skilled in anti-miasmatic prescribing dips deeper into the case, and applies an agent that has a deeper and closer relationship with the prevented life-force. The results are always better.

A knowledge of all miasmatic phenomena would be a complete knowledge of all that is known as disease. Hahnemann discovered the miasms due to the fact that these ailments kept coming back, year after year. Even with the correct remedy being given, there was no permanent cure. His proof of the existence was the persistence of these chronic diseases, constantly repeating themselves. The conditions that would modify a miasm in a person's body would be factors, like climate, and peculiar and physical character of the person it is in, mental delays, excesses or abuses in life, in diet, passions, habits and various customs. Allopathic doctors have put names on various diseases such as jaundice, dropsy, leucorrhoea, haemorrhoids, eczema, asthma, rheumatism, herpes, to name a few. Hahnemann considered all these based from the same beginnings.

During the days of Hahnemann, the homoeopathic world was divided into two groups:

1. Those who believed in miasms.
2. Those who did not.

In the early days of this theory very few of Hahnemann's pupils accepted this theory wholeheartedly. There were others like Hering who became converts with experience. There were still others like Richard Hughes who never believed it, and even went on to call this theory of miasms, Hahnemann's greatest mistake.

Later, with the rise of Kent and the advent of microbiology and bacteriology, even the believers split into two groups:

1. Those who believed Hahnemann's miasms were nothing but bacteria and viruses.
2. Those who believed in the spiritual nature of the miasms.

Dr Hering, Richard Hughes, Stuart Close, G Boericke, Margaret Tyler, P Speight, BK Sarkar, Harimohan Chaudhary—all have favoured the concept that miasms are bacteria, or originate from bacterial diseases. Some of these people even went on to call Hahnemann, the Father of Bacteriology, because his description of miasms was so similar to the bacteria at many places. Others like Kent, JH Allen, J Paterson, H.A. Roberts, etc., strongly believed in the non-material nature of the miasms. They described miasms as a dyscrasia, a state and a predisposition. Kent even went on to say, "Psora is the underlying cause, the primitive or primary disorder of the human race... it goes to the very primitive wrong of the human race, the very first sickness of the human race, that is, the spiritual sickness...."

If one goes through the various works of Hahnemann closely, one will realise that he has used the term 'miasm' in different senses at different places. Maybe he himself was confused. On one hand, he was talking about the spiritual vital force and its dynamic derangement as the cause of all diseases; on the other hand, he was well aware that there was something material (contagion) in acute diseases, like cholera and typhus, and chronic diseases like syphilis and gonorrhoea. We need to understand that he was trying to understand the cause of disease without the aid of any microscopes. He was just relying on his keen observation, and apart from his observation, there was nothing much to support him. Developing a whole classification of diseases was a marvellous work done by him. He had his own limitations and the work he did within those limitations is indeed extraordinary.

Various Theories

By the late 1790's, Hahnemann had realised that syphilis was an infectious blood disease that could mask itself with the symptoms of many different illnesses. Early in his career, he made a special preparation called *Mercurius Solubis Hahnemanni* that was the standard treatment for syphilis throughout Europe. He soon found that mercury in homoeopathic potency worked much better on syphilis than the crude poisonous form, and he recorded several permanent cures.

At this time, there were four major theories about diseases that spread in an infectious manner:

1. Miasm as a foul, gaseous exhalation
2. The theory of the animalcule
3. The zymotic theory
4. The theory of spontaneous generation

The followers of the spontaneous generation theory believed that germs appeared whenever the conditions were right for the development without the need for reproduction. In some sense, this is true as, where did the 'first germ' come from?

The zymotist suggested that certain substances called 'zymes' that were inert outside the body could lie dormant until the internal terrain made it possible for them to multiply, and caused specific diseases. The observations of the zymotists are very similar to the activities of viral material in the human body. The term 'zymotic' can be found in the old homoeopathic literature and is a rubric in the general section of Kent's *Repertory*.

Hahnemann synthesised the ideas of the animalcule and zymes, and redefined the Hippocratic term 'miasma' to express the constitutional derangements caused by parasitic infections. He carefully separated the self-limiting acute miasms from the syndromes of long-lasting diseases, and started to develop a special *Materia Medica* and repertory for the treatment of the chronic miasms. Therefore, in Hahnemannian homoeopathy, the word 'miasm' means the effects of micro organisms on the vital force, including the symptoms that are transmitted to the following generations. These chronic miasms are capable of producing degenerative illnesses, auto-immune diseases, and lead the organism toward immuno-deficiency disorders.

Three Chronic Miasms

Hahnemann noticed that each of the chronic diseases has three phases:

1. A primary stage
2. A latent stage
3. A secondary or tertiary state

The effects of these miasms were then passed from one generation to the next generation by inheritance, and caused predispositions to certain disease syndromes. The three chronic miasms that Hahnemann introduced in 1828 were called psora (the itch miasm), sycosis (the gonorrhal miasm) and syphilis (the chancre miasm). He published his miasmic theory long before the presence of germs was widely accepted, so most practitioners found it hard to understand such a sophisticated theory of contagion.

From the time of Hippocrates healers conjectured about the possibility of invisible organisms causing diseases but Hahnemann founded the modern concept of infection. In fact, homoeopathic pathology is still more advanced than its modern allopathic counterpart which still does not understand the effects of the miasmic processes or their inherited constitutional syndromes.

Hahnemann published *The Chronicle Disease* in 1828, and introduced the idea of categorising deep acting remedies by the chronic miasms. This is an integral part of our homoeopathic heritage, and should not be forgotten if we are to cure the most complex forms of chronic disease.

Why is it necessary for a homoeopath to know the chronic miasms? Some might say as long as one prescribes according to the law of similars he cures his cases. The important factor here is "as long as he selects the most similar remedy as possible". The fact is we cannot find the most similar remedy possible unless we understand the phenomena of the acting miasm. The true *similia* is always based on the existing miasm. It makes the difference between fighting the disease in the dark and in bright light when one knows the underlying principle that fathers the phenomena. If one has no knowledge of the laws of action and reaction, how can we watch the progress of a case without a definite knowledge of the disease forces (miasms) with their mysterious and persistent progressions. So, if we can know nothing about the traits and characteristics of our enemy, it is impossible to wage a war against the disease.

The chronic diseases are held to be responsible for all diseases of chronic nature, and to form the foundation or basis for all diseases in general. This latter aspect was then to receive considerable amplification from Kent. Kent was also able to identify those remedies that relate to each miasm.

Though now generally accepted by most homoeopaths without question, at that time the theory was generally greeted with disbelief and derision from all but the most devoted followers. This can be explained in part by the primitive nature of medical science at that time, which was not really very willing to accommodate any theory for the origin of disease, least of all such a grand and all-embracing one.

The theory suggests that if 100 per cent of all diseases is miasmic, then 85 per cent is due to the primary and atavistic miasm that Hahnemann called psora. The remaining 15 per cent of all diseases he held to be either syphilitic or sycotic, being derived from suppressed syphilis or suppressed gonorrhoea. Hahnemann, unlike Kent, later attached no moral dimension whatsoever to the sexual nature of the latter two miasms. Kent, of course, emphasised this a great deal, which is hardly surprising in the somewhat puritanical atmosphere of nineteenth century small town America.

Each of the chronic miasms have their own characteristic signs that are an integral part of the totality of the symptoms. For example, psora tends to produce irritation, inflammation and hyper-sensitivity; sycosis produces infiltrations, over-growth and indurations; syphilis tends toward granulation, degeneration and ulceration.

In the preface of Charles Hempel's translation of *The Organon,* Constantine Hering recorded that late in his life, Hahnemann made further discoveries and developed a new aspect of the theory of psora with the introduction of a new miasm he called pseudo-psora. Hering wrote, "Hahnemann distinguishes the venereal miasms as syphilis and sycosis; and also subdivides psora with pseudo-psora." This pseudo-psora tends to produce fibrosis, tuberculosis and suppuration.

Hahnemann's miasmic theory now contained two venereal and two non-venereal miasms that produced lifelong chronic diseases. The two non-venereal miasms are psora (the itch disease) and pseudo-psora (the tubercle disease). The two venereal miasms are sycosis (the fig-wart diseases) and syphilis (the chancere disease). Hahnemann noticed that some cases that appeared to be psora did not depend exclusively on an external skin eruption for their development. He observed that this disease was infectious in nature and possessed primary, latent and secondary symptoms as well as inherited aspects. He decided that it was caused by a miasmic agent with a distinct etiology, so he separated its symptoms from psora, and made a new classification called the pseudo-psora, the tuberculosis miasm. All of these miasms may be acquired through a primary infection, or their effects can be experienced through heredity.

It is sometimes thought that Hahnemann taught that all long-lasting diseases are caused by chronic miasms. This is not the total picture.

In *The Organon,* he mentions three classifications of long-lasting disease:

1. Those caused by continuing stress factors (disorders upheld by maintaining causes which, by their nature, are not necessarily true chronic disorders).
2. Those caused by drug toxicity and faulty treatment (physician caused).
3. Those caused by infectious miasms (naturally caused).

Physical Expressions of the Miasms

The mind and body work together as a unit, and the disturbances are expressed in both spheres.

Psoric miasm: reaction of body on exposure to environmental stimuli to one's surroundings like noise, light and smell, producing functional disturbances like headache, nausea, and discomfort. Psora tends to make the organism toxic, the skin unhealthy, and perverts the functions of the digestive and eliminative organs.

Pseudo-psora: tends to produce pipe-stem bones; narrow chests, sunken cheeks and sparkling eyes.

Sycotic miasm: hypersensitive reaction to something specific arising from a deficiency of the normal response like tumours, allergies, keloids. A deficient feeling gives rise to an increased attempt to repair the fault. Sycosis tends to cause heavy bones, water retention, overgrowth of tissue and slow metabolism.

Syphilitic miasm: not manageable, finding destruction like gangrene and ulceration. Body and mind destroy themselves. Syphilis tends to cause congenital defects, asymmetrical long structure, deformed teeth and the classic bull-dog face.

The following are the personality and temperament types.

Psoric miasm: highs and lows; struggling with the outside world; becomes transparent at times of stress; lack of confidence; constant anxiety feelings; fear like he can't do it; insecurity; anxiety about the future but always having hope, mentally alert. He is full of pseudo-scientific, philosophical, political, religious ideas. He is self-expressive, talkative, self-deceptive and may think he is full of genius but seems foolish and impractical to others.

Sycotic miasm: secretive; hides his weakness; tense; constantly covering up situations; fixed habits; suspicious; jealous; forgetful. He is pessimistic, a hard realist, sceptical, and has self-hidden disgust.

Pseudo-psora: romantic; erotic; social; extrovert, cosmopolitan; erratic; optimistic; yet dissatisfied and always wants to change jobs, places, mates, etc.

Syphilitic miasm: strong; pessimistic view on life; cannot modify what is wong; give up or destroy, no point in trying to adjust; sudden impulsive violence directed at himself or others, dictational rigid ideas; mental paralysis; mentally dull, suicidal tendency, stupid; stubborn and homicidal. He has a mixture of madness and genius with a deep sense of irony that leads to obsession with death and destruction. He becomes guilty, self-destructive, and ends in idiocy, insanity or suicide.

The general nature of the miasm manifests in the following way:

Psoric miasm: itching; burning; inflammation leading to congestion; philosopher; selfish; restless; weak; has fears. He has sensations of itchiness; crawling; tickling and burning.

Pseudo-psoric miasm: the pains are neuralgic, sharp, piercing, twisting, stitching.

Sycotic miasm: over-production of growth like warts; condylomata; fibrous tissue; disease of internal organs, pelvis and sexual organs. The pains are sudden, intense, spasmodic, crampy and colicky.

Syphilitic miasm: destructive; disorder everywhere; ulceration; fissures; deformities; suicidal; depressed; memory diminished. The pains seem lacking for the conditions present, or are deep, aching, agonising, and especially more at night.

The dermatological symptoms of the miasms are as follows.

Psoric miasm: dirty, dry, itching without pus or discharge; burning; scaly eruptions, eczema; cracks in hands and feet; sweat profuse, especially during sleep; being offensive. The skin is unhealthy, every little injury becomes infected, and the lesions are itchy without pus.

Pseudo-sporic miasm: the skin of the pseudopsora is translucent, fine, smooth, bruises easily, and its lesions bleed easily exuding excessive pus.

Sycotic miasm: warty; moles; unnatural thickening of skin; herpes; scars; nails thick and irregular; oily skin that is corrugated and oozing; disturbed pigment in patches. The skin also has flecks, growths, dark discolourations with overgrowth of hair.

Syphilitic miasm: ulcers; boils; discharge of fluids; offensive pus slow to heal; leprosy; copper-coloured eruptions aggravated by heat of bed; spoon-shaped thin nails that tear easily; putrid gangrene. There are eruptions that do not itch but have a tendency towards ulceration.

In *The Organon,* Hahnemann states, "The true, natural chronic diseases are those that arise from a chronic miasm; when left to themselves, improper treatment, go on to increase, growing worse, and torment the patient to the end of his life." In his *Chronic Diseases,* he describes how using antisporic medicines on the psora miasm would enable a practitioner to cure effectively.

Psora has passed on through hundreds of generations of people, and produced an innumerable variety of defects, injuries, derangements and sufferings. Chronic miasms are very hidden, and the symptoms are much more difficult to be ascertained.

The miasmatic clinicals are as follows:

Psoric miasm: acidity; burning; cancer; sarcoma; constipation; epilepsy; flatulence; hoarseness; itching of skin; leprosy; burning of spinal cord; watery discharge from nose and eyes.

Sycotic miasm: abortion, acne without pus, angina pectoris, anaemia; appendicitis; whooping cough; colic; pelvic and sexual organ diseases; piles; prostatis; nephritis; gout; arthritis; dry asthma; dysmenorrhoea; herpes; rheumatism; warts; urinary ailments.

Syphilitis miasm: discharges putrefaction; blindness; boils in veins and over bones; carcinomas; fistula; fungal infection of extremities; gangrene; hypertension; bone marrow inflammation; insanity due to depression; leucorrhoea; rheumatism of long bones; skin disease with ooze and pus; sore throat; history of abortions;

sterility; early death; cardiac arrests; suicidal deaths; cancer; tuberculosis; ulcers of ear and nose and urinary organs.

Types of Miasms

There are two types of miasms that affect us directly. They are inherited miasms and acquired miasms.

1. *Inherited miasms*

The inheritance of miasms is not genetic, and actually takes place because the vital force of parents is tainted by such states, as observed with mother and father at the time of conception. Miasms are seen to be transmitted to the offspring. It is not the pathology which shows the miasm but the state, the characteristics in that individual, keeping with the mental and physical state. The three combined reflect the miasm. A diseased state is usually a combination of miasms with its main focus on one miasm.

It is important to perceive each miasmatic state of the remedy in order to understand the diseased state, because then we become aware of how a person perceives and reacts to his surroundings, how he perceives himself, and how he reacts when things become unmanageable and stressful.

2. *Acquired miasms*

Not only do we inherit miasms but we acquire them from our environment during a lifetime, because we live in a toxic surrounding. There are literally thousands of miasms in the polluted world of today, for example, radiation. We are exposed to radiation from X-rays in hospitals and dentists' surgeries, aeroplane flights. It is also found in irradiated foods. Nuclear accidents and bomb-testing spin the radiation out to the earth's poles by the action of rotation of the earth, thereby affecting everyone, no matter where they are.

Acquired miasms become inherited miasms in the next generation through the birth process. An indication that miasms and resonances do exist was shown to us by Hahnemann about 200 years ago. He used the positive or beneficial resonances of homoeopathy to remove the negative resonances from patients' connective tissues and subtle bodies, thus effecting a cure from their illnesses.

Elimination of Miasms

Today, there is a way of removing or eliminating all of the pollutants and miasms, using the modality called isopathy. This is a detox programme par excellence that uses a sequential toxic removal system which John Godwin has called the TPO or Toxic Pecking Order. This procedure involves the use of a specialised machine known as the EAV machine.

It is now recognised that all matter has its own individual resonance or vibration. With this in mind, the use of a vial of the homoeopathic miasm or poison in conjunction with an EAV machine enables us to measure miasms or poisons present in the physical and subtle bodies. A homoeopathic/isopathic remedy that is an exact copy of the vibration of the original miasm or poison is then administered to the patient. These remedies are potentised so that, with their positive resonance, they eliminate the negative resonance of the pollutant/poison/miasm.

Miasms in the Modern World

After Hahnemann, many homoeopaths have suggested that, since miasms are disease syndromes, there can be more miasms than psora, syphilis and sycosis. The concept is to look for diseases which leave a diseased state in the body even after apparent recovery, especially after suppression. In this regard, the following miasms have been proposed so far:

1. Tubercular by J.H. Allen
2. Vaccinosis by Dr Burnett
3. Cancer
4. Malaria by R. Sankaran
5. Ringworm by R. Sankaran
6. Typhoid by R. Sankaran
7. Leprosy by R. Sankaran
8. Smallpox

The understanding and approach of those who have put forward newer miasms are varied and at odds with Hahnemann's ideas. As a result, the world of miasms has become more chaotic.

How Do You Treat Miasms?

Miasms are integrated into our innermost being since thousands of years in the ancestry. Although they are not difficult to correct with homoeopathy, they are not always wiped out in a single blow.

Homoeopaths have shown how miasms exist in various layers in the body, and that as we work at correcting disease and building good health, it is like peeling away the layers of an onion. These layers are like overlays as seen in global maps demonstrating how global shifts and changes in boundaries of countries have taken place over time and warfare.

Treating miasms can cause extreme change in one's health. Generally, these changes can cause a wonderfully euphoric experience, and when intense cleansing occurs, there may be a temporary discomfort from the eliminative process. Some of the commonly experienced cleansing symptoms may include emotional releases, skin eruptions, itching, fever, fatigue, bowel movement changes, breathing changes and various forms of pain. These symptoms, although temporary and not harmful to the body, can be severe at times. While the body is orchestrating the healing process, it will not harm or cause any permanent damage to it. The healing is not always comfortable or convenient, but it is essential for healing and restoration of one's health.

While using the miasm formulas, it is best to monitor patients closely for there is a 60 per cent chance of experiencing some form of cleansing. This way, while experiencing these symptoms, the patients will understand the need for cleansing and eradicating the miasms. This helps them to correct their present disease(s), and also to prevent diseases in the future, both in their future offspring and themselves. Before treating the patient, some explanation about the treatment will make a big difference in the attitude of the patient when he goes through a cleansing crisis.

When treating a new patient, it would be advisable to address the primary symptoms with symptoms-specific formulas first, along with detox and drainage formulas. This will help strengthen and restore the natural healing and eliminative functions first so that the homoeopath can deal better with deeper issues of the miasms later.

Miasms are great to use when patients:
1. Don't respond to homoeopathic treatment.
2. Don't respond to other natural treatment.
3. Reach plateaus where they seem to level off in their health enhancement.
4. Continue to have recurrences with the same problem.

Miasms have a tendency to show up periodically throughout the healing processes over years. Even miasms that did not show up previously in testing show up later on in the treatment programme as more of the layers of the disease have been peeled away. Either the same miasm treatment or different miasm treatments will commonly be needed periodically over our lives. It is likely that almost everyone has at least one miasm. Many people have more than one.

Treatment with a miasm formula may last for a few days to a few months at a time. Dosages can vary from two to six times per day. Again, bio-feedback or reflex response tests are the best guide to dosage, length of treatment, and when to repeat treatment for maximum results.

The Theory of Latent Psora

"Psora is that most ancient, most universal, most destructive, and yet most misapprehended chronic miasmatic disease which, for many thousands of years, has disfigured and tortured mankind... and become the mother of all the thousands of incredibly various chronic diseases..." (Hahnemann, *Chronic Diseases*).

Kent, in his *Lectures,* then greatly enlarged upon the theory, proposing that psora was the foundation of all other illnesses, without which mankind would be pure and healthy, both in mind and body, thus regarded psora as being equated with the 'Fall of Man' and with original sinfulness. He portrayed psora in this highly moralistic light as also being the foundation of the sexual miasms that came later.

To discover the true psoric remedies, we must add together the remedies listed in the *Repertory* for a range of psoric conditions. This means checking carefully all the symptoms and repertorising for all of them, gradually building up a master list of remedies that fit psoric conditions. This exercise was highly recommended by Kent as a sure way of fixing in the mind the remedies of a particular miasm. It is also an excellent introduction to the miasms generally, and is good for revision purposes. With computer programmes, this task becomes a lot easier than it was in Kent's or Hahnemann's days.

Since the 1950's, it has been claimed that tuberculosis and cancer have developed into miasms in their own right, most probably as offshoots of what Hahnemann termed as the 'hydra-headed psora miasm' in his *Chronic Diseases*. Fifty-nine symptoms and major conditions were selected and repertorised, using Kent's *Repertory*. The symptoms were as follows.

TB	Swollen tonsils
TB incipient	Swollen axillary glands
TB pituitous	Buboes
Scabies	Goitre
Psoriasis	Tooth decay
Dandruff	Deafness
Hair loss	Insanity
Leprosy	Asthma
Cancer	Liver
Cancer Lupus	Haemorrhoids
Leukaemia	Itching anus
Diabetes	Offensive stools
Cataract	Varicosities
Blindness	Numbness of Limbs
Long-sightedness	Chilblains
Short-sightedness	Sweaty feet
Lack of reaction	Offensive foot sweats
Takes cold easily	Halitosis (nasal crusts)
Swollen neck glands	Perianal moisture
Indurated neck glands	Hay fever
Foul flatus	Scrotal swelling
Cracking joints	Dysuria
Worms	Eczema
Ulcers on legs	Herpetic skin eruptions

Ringworm   Crusty skin eruptions
Haemoptysis   Pleurisy
Stomach ulcers   Swollen inguinal glands
Jaundice   Malaria
Smallpox

These symptoms were chosen as they are in the list given by Hahnemann as of 'latent psora', or they are major diseases of modern life. Hahnemann assumed that were derived from suppressed scabies, leprosy or plague. They are disorders mentioned in Hahnemann's *Chronic Diseases* as often being the products of suppressed itch, or they are skin disorders in their own right. To an extent, one major justification for choosing these symptoms is that they have all increased during this century, which many take to be a confirmation of the psora doctrine.

11

The Organon of Medicine

Stuart Close, the late professor of homoeopathic philosophy, New York Homoeopathic Medical College, states, "Dynamism, the Vital Force, Potentiation and the Infinitesimal Dose: Around these three subjects have centred the hottest controversies and the most mordant criticisms in the history of homoeopathy; and these are the newly treated subjects in the Sixth Edition of *The Organon.* " He goes on to add, "To Hahnemann belongs the honour of having been the first physician to connect biology and psychology with physics in a practical system of medicinal therapeutics, and to give an impulse to studies in biodynamics which has gained momentum continuously ever since" (*The Genius of Homoeopathy: Lectures and Essays on Homoeopathic Philosophy*).

The Organon is the work on which homoeopathy is based. Five editions were brought out by Hahnemann while still alive, while the sixth one was brought out decades after his death.

Hahnemann's work was ridiculed in the beginning because it did not conform to current medical thinking. Over years of experience his works gradually became accepted and credited even with the ruling elite. When the sixth edition was published after his death, ironically it was the homoeopaths who refused to accept some of the newer principles and ideas that he presented.

Hahnemann almost exclusively used LM potencies in later years of his life which were recorded in his sixth edition. He declared that the LM potency, a dilution of a 3C in 500 drops of water, eliminated or reduced aggravations, especially for sensitive individuals.

Since homoeopaths were successful using C and X potencies, they were reluctant to accept the success of LM potencies.

When some found greater success with newer potencies, these potencies too got established in the homoeopathic system of medicine. Today all three types of potencies are used, each with effectiveness for specific circumstances.

The sixth edition contains 291 paragraphs or aphorisms, the first 70 relating to the theoretical components, and the rest with practical ones.

The following are the aphorisms given briefly:

1, 2: The sole mission of the physician is to cure rapidly, gently, permanently. (Note: Not to construct theoretical systems, nor to attempt to explain phenomena.)

3, 4: He must investigate what is to be cured in disease and know what is curative in the various medicines, in order to be able to adapt the latter to the former, and must also understand how to preserve the health of human beings.

Paragraphs 5 to 18 centre around the knowledge of diseases, its causes, types, history, the need for removal and the means to accomplish it.

5: Attention to exciting and fundamental clauses and other circumstances, helps to cure.

6: For the physician, the disease consists only of the totality of its symptoms.

7: Whilst paying attention to those circumstances (para 5), the physician needs only to remove the totality of the symptoms in order to cure the disease.

8: If all the symptoms be eradicated, the disease is always cured internally also.

9: During health, a spiritual power (vital force) animates the organism and keeps it in harmonious order.

10:_ Without this animating, spirit-like power, the organism is dead.

11: In disease, the vital force only is primarily morbidly deranged, and expresses its sufferings (the internal change) by abnormal sensations and functions of the organism.

12: By the disappearance of the totality of the symptoms by the cure, the affection of the vital force, that is to say, the whole internal and external morbid state is also removed.

13: To regard those diseases that are not surgical as a peculiar distinct thing residing in the human frame is an absurdity which has rendered allopathy so pernicious.

14: Everything of a morbid nature that is curable makes itself known to the physician by disease symptoms.

15: The affection of the diseased vital force and the disease symptoms thereby produced, constitute an inseparable whole—they are one and the same.

16: It is only by the spiritual principles of morbific noxae that our spirit-like vital force can become ill; and in like manner, only by the spirit-like (dynamic) operation of medicines that it can be again restored to health.

17: The practitioner, therefore, only needs to take away the totality of the disease signs, and he has removed the entire disease.

18: The totality of the symptoms is the only indication, the only guide to the selection of a remedy.

Paragraphs 19 to 27 deal with the knowledge of medicines, their power to alter a state of ill health, their power, to provide a proving by dosing a healthy individual, their curative principles, their similarities to a diseased state, aggravations from dosing, their ability to create an artificial state in a healthy person, the complete eradication of symptoms with the medicines, and theory related to it, their strength and the power of the medicine to specific symptoms.

19: The alteration of the state of health in diseases (the disease symptoms) cannot be cured by the medicines otherwise than in so far as the latter have the power of also producing alterations in man's health.

20: This power of medicines to alter the state of the health can only be ascertained by their effects on healthy persons.

21: The morbid symptoms that medicines produce in healthy individuals are the only factor wherefrom we can learn their disease-curing power.

22: If experience show that by medicines that manifest similar symptoms to the disease the latter would be most certainly and permanently cured, we must select for the cure medicines with similar symptoms; but should it show that the disease is most certainly and permanently cured by opposite medicinal symptoms, we must choose for the cure medicines with opposite symptoms.

23: By opposite medicinal symptoms (antipathic treatment) persisting disease symptoms are not cured.

24, 25: The other retaining method of treatment, the homoeopathic, by means of medicines with similar symptoms, is the only one that experience shows to be always salutary.

26: This is dependent on the therapeutic law of nature that a weaker dynamic affection in the living organism is permanently extinguished by one that is very similar to and stronger than it, only differs from it in kind.

27: The curative power of medicines, therefore, depends on the symptoms they have similar to the disease of the healthy.

Paragraphs 28 to 70 focus on the choice of the remedy and its administration.

28, 29:   Attempt to explain this therapeutic law of nature.

30-33:   The human body is much more disposed to let its state of health be altered by medicinal forces than by natural disease.

34, 35:   The correctness of the homoeopathic therapeutic law is shown in the want of success attending every unhomoeopathic treatment of a long-standing disease, and in this also, that two natural diseases meeting together in the body, if they be dissimilar to each other, do not remove or cure one another.

36:   The older disease existing in the body, if it be equally as strong or stronger, keeps away from the patient a new dissimilar disease.

37:   Thus under, unhomoeopathic treatment that is not violent, chronic diseases remain as they were.

38:   A new, stronger disease, attacking an individual already ill, suppresses only, as long as it lasts, the old disease that is dissimilar to it, already present in the body, but never removes it.

39:   It is just in this way that violent treatment with allopathic drugs does not cure a chronic disease, but suppresses it only as long as the action of the powerful medicines, which are unable to excite any symptoms, similar to the disease lasts; after that, the chronic disease makes its appearance as bad as or worse than before.

40:   Or the new disease, after having long acted on the body, joins the old one that is dissimilar to it, and thence arises a double (complex) disease; neither of these two dissimilar diseases removes the other.

41:   In the course of nature, it is not seldom that two dissimilar diseases meet in the same organism, but this happens much more frequently in the ordinary employment of powerful, inappropriate (allopathic) medicine, associates itself with the old natural disease, which is similar to (and therefore not curable by) the former, and the chronic patient now becomes doubly diseased.

42: These diseases that thus complicate one another take, on account of their dissimilarity, each the place in the organism suited for it.

43, 44: But quite otherwise is it on the accession of a stronger disease to a pre-existing one similar to it; in that case the latter will be removed and cured by the former.

45: Explanation of this phenomenon.

46: Instances of chronic diseases being cured by the accidental accession of another similar but stronger disease.

47-49: In cases where diseases come together in the course of nature, it is only one that displays similar symptoms that can remove and cure the other, a dissimilar disease can never do this; this should teach the physician what kind of medicines he can certainly cure with, namely, with homoeopathic ones alone.

50: Nature has but few diseases to send to the homoeopathic relief of other diseases, and remedial agents are accompanied by many inconveniences.

51: On the other hand, the physician has innumerable remedial agents, possessing great advantages over those.

52: There are but two chief methods of cure, the homoeopathic and the allopathic, which are exact opposites, they cannot approach each other or unite.

53: The homoeopathic is based on an infallible law of nature, and proves itself as the only excellent one.

54: The allopathic appeared in many differing systems following each other, all terming themselves rational methods of cure. This method saw in diseases only morbid matter which were classified and created a *Materia Medica* based on conjectures and compound prescriptions.

55, 56: The allopathic physicians possess in their hurtful method of treatment nothing but palliatives which still may retain the confidence of patients.

57: The antipathic or enantiopathic or palliative method treats a single symptom of a disease with a remedy of opposite action.

58: This antipathic procedure is not defective merely because it is directed against a single symptom of the disease only, but also because in perishing ailments, after it produces a short apparent ameliorations, real aggravation ensues.

59: Injurious effects of some antipathic modes of treatment.

60: Increasing the dose at every repetition of a palliative never cures a chronic affection, but does more harm.

61: Whenever physicians ought to have inferred the utility of an opposite and only good mode of treatment, to wit, the homoeopathic.

62: The reason for the injurious nature of the palliative, and for the sole efficacy of the homoeopathic employment of medicines.

63: Depends upon the difference between the primary action that takes place under the influence of every medicine, and the reaction or secondary action subsequently effected by the living organism (the vital force).

64: Explanation of the primary and secondary actions.

65: Examples of both.

66: From the smallest homoeopathic doses of medicine employed in treatment, the secondary action of the vital force merely shows itself in the restoration of the balance of health.

67: These truths explain the salutary character of the homoeopathic treatment, as also the perversity of the antipathic (palliative) method.

68: How is the efficacy of the homoeopathic system proved by these truths?

69: How is the hurtfulness of the antipathic treatment proved by these truths?

70: Short summary of the homoeopathic system of medicine.

Paragraphs 71 to 102 begin with the practical aspects of homoeopathy, and explain how a practitioner can determine what is important in case-taking. Acute and chronic diseases, vital energy and miasms are touched upon.

71: The three points necessary for curing:
   a. the investigation of the disease.
   b. the investigation of the effects of the medicines.
   c. their appropriate employment.

72: General survey of diseases—acute, chronic.

73: Acute diseases that attack single individuals, sporadic, epidemic, acute miasms.

74: The worst kinds of chronic diseases are those produced by the unskilfulness of allopathic physicians. The most allopathic debilitating treatment of Brosseau.

75: These are the most incurable.

76: It is only when the vital force is still sufficiently powerful that the injury can then be repaired, often only after a long time, if the original disease be at the same time homoeopathically eradicated.

152: For those with numerous striking symptoms a homoeopathic remedy can be more certainly found.

153: What kind of symptoms ought one chiefly to attend to in the choice of a remedy?

154: A remedy as homoeopathic as it is possible to be cured without much disturbance.

155: Cause of the freedom from disturbance of such cures.

156: Cause of the slight exceptions to this.

157-160: The medicinal disease very similar, but somewhat superior in strength, to the original disease, termed also homoeopathic aggravation.

161: In chronic (psoric) diseases the homoeopathic aggravations from (antisporic) homoeopathic medicines occur during a period of several days, from time to time.

162-171: Rules for treatment when the supply of known medicines is too small to allow a perfect homoeopathic remedy to be discovered.

172-184: Rules for the treatment of diseases with too few symptoms: one-sided diseases.

185-203: Treatment of diseases with local symptoms; their external treatment is always injurious.

204, 205: All chronic affections and diseases properly so called (that are not merely produced and maintained by a bad mode of living) must be cured only from within, by the homoeopathic medicines appropriate for the miasm that lies at their root.

206: Preliminary investigation of the miasm that lies at their root, of the simple miasm or its complications with a second (or even with a third).

207: Inquiry into the treatments previously employed.

208, 209: The other preliminary inquiries necessary for the apprehension of the morbid picture of the chronic disease.

287:    Mineral magnet.

288, 289:   Animal magnetism. Mesmerism.

290:    Massage.

291:    Water baths as remedial agents according to their temperature.

The Organon of Medicine was Samuel Hahnemann's magnum opus. His formulation of the fundamental law of healing, called the law of similars, states that a patient will be cured by a medicinal substance producing the same disease symptoms in a healthy person. First published in 1810, and subsequently revised six times, the *Organon* has remained the one essential cornerstone of homoeopathy, the ultimate authority on its doctrine and practice.

One can find distinct changes between the fifth and sixth editions. The latter contains rewritten paragraphs, additions and deletions, new processes and possibly unauthorised editing. Certain external applications of medicines are also discussed.

12

Homoeopathic Provings

The practice of homoeopathy is a three-part process. It involves learning about the patient's disease, learning about the remedies and finding a match between them. The first and last of these processes are quite well known, but the process of finding out about remedies is not often written about or discussed. This process is called the proving of remedies.

Proving is the process associated with the homoeopathic method of testing substances in order to establish their 'symptom pictures'. In other words, a homoeopathic proving is the method by which the profile of a homoeopathic remedy is determined. Constantine Hering sums it up very well

> "Proving is a most wonderful, thing like the world has never known its like. We suffer, and we enjoy it; we sacrifice a little of our comfort, and gain years of strength by it; we go to school to learn, and we increase the certainty of the healing art. At the same time, to probe drugs is of all other ways the very best, the nearest and the easiest to learn to master our *Materia Medica*. It is the way to learn, to observe the art of arts, the principal one on which all others are based.

Provings are carried out in a number of ways, depending on the group which is conducting the trial. This usually involves following Samuel Hahnemann's strict protocol, but may extend to a person taking the remedy and meditating on the effects. It should however be noted that most authoritative provings are done following a strict method, laid down in Jeremy Sherr's book entitled *The Dynamics and Methodology of Homoeopathic Provings*. All symptoms—physical, emotional and mental—are noted in detail, then gathered in a systematic way, common themes noted, collated and published in the homoeopathic *Materia Medica*.

Hahnemann's Provings

Provings, or pathogeneses with the various substances, were always done on healthy subjects, and all reactions were recorded. The first compilation of provings was published in 1810 as *The Organon* (The Art of Healing) by Hahnemann. Other physicians have continued his work, and today's homoeopathic *Materia Medica* makes the records of years of provings available to homoeopathic physicians.

To attempt determine which homoeopathic remedies would be best for various ailments, Hahnemann and others got engaged in a series of provings. In what can be viewed as early clinical trials of natural substances, Hahnemann and others, self-administered pharmacologically active doses of many different substances, then carefully recorded the symptoms that resulted, in the *Materia Medica*.

These provings were based on Hahnemann's early study of cinchona bark. In 1790, he took several doses of cinchona which was used to treat malaria. Symptoms of trembling and cold limbs, heart palpitations, etc., were noted. The symptoms returned with each subsequent dose. He recorded that cinchona bark was effective against malaria, because it could produce similar symptoms in healthy people. This led to testing additional drugs, not previously known to be effective, to find their potential use as remedies. Between 1811 and 1821, Hahnemann carried out provings of many homoeopathic medicines, and published the results.

Hahnemann and his followers conducted the provings in which they administered herbs, minerals and other substances to healthy people, including themselves, and kept detailed records of what they observed. Later, these recordings were compiled into lengthy reference books called *Materia Medica* which are used to match a patient's symptoms with a corresponding drug.

Hahnemann declared that diseases represent a disturbance in the body's ability to heal itself, and that only a small stimulus is needed to begin the healing process. He also claimed that chronic diseases were manifestations of a suppressed itch (psora), a kind of miasm or evil spirit. At first he used small doses of accepted medications. But later he used enormous dilutions and theorised that the smaller the dose, the more powerful the effect a motion referred to commonly as the 'Law of infinitesimal'. That, of course, is just the opposite of the dose-response relationship that pharmacologists have demonstrated. Hahnemann states,

> There is, therefore, no other possible way in which the peculiar effects of medicines on the health of individuals can be accurately ascertained...than to administer the several medicines experimentally, in moderate doses, to healthy persons, in order to ascertain what changes, symptoms and signs of their influence each individually produces on the health of the body and of the mind; that is to say, what disease elements they are able and tend to produce, since, as has been demonstrated, all the curative powers of medicines lies in this power they possess of changing the state of man's health, and is revealed by observation of the latter.

Hahnemann felt that the best proving was done on oneself. Since the proving is based on self-observation, Hahnemann cautions that the person doing the proving must be trustworthy, intelligent, and have keen observational skills. Some provings were taken from literature, particularly where poisonings from a known agent produced a specific pattern of symptoms or lesions.

Hahnemann stressed with his own provings that homoeopaths should add to the *Materia Medica* with their provings too. He states in his *The Organon* (sixth edition),

> At first, about forty years ago, I was the only person who made the provings of the pure powders of medicines the most important of my occupations. Since then I have been assisted in this by some young men, who instituted experiments on themselves, and whose observations I have critically revised. Following these, some genuine work of this kind was done by a few others. But

what shall we not be able to effect in the way of curing in the whole extent of the infinitely large domain of disease, when numbers of accurate and trustworthy observers shall have rendered their services in enriching this, the only true *Materia Medica* by careful experiments on themselves! The healing art will then come near the mathematical sciences in certainty.

What Proving Involves

A proving typically involves 20 volunteers taking six doses of the remedy over two days. If symptoms occur, then no further doses should be taken. During this time, for some time after, each prover keeps a proving diary, recording all mental, physical and emotional symptoms that are experienced during the proving.

At the end of the proving period the master prover will collate the symptoms from the diaries, excluding those symptoms which have been demonstrated to be symptoms that the prover experienced, before the proving commenced. This part of the process can be quite time-consuming. Finally, the proving is published in its entirety.

In order to give a full remedy picture, it is normal for provers to take the remedy at a range of potencies. A more recent development occasionally involved having some of the participants in a trial take a placebo. The symptoms recorded by these provers are compared to the symptoms recorded by the other provers in order to aid the process of deciding which symptoms are caused by the remedy. It should be noted that in some, such 'placebo-controlled' provings may not qualify as either randomised or double-blind trials, since the participants are not randomised and the master prover is routinely aware of who is on placebo. In most modern, well-conducted provings even the master proving is not aware of who is on placebo, and may therefore be legitimately regarded as double blind. A curious fact is that in some instances, the provers on placebo have been observed to produce symptoms similar to those who are taking the remedy, a fact which some homoeopaths attribute to field effects or energetic resonance.

Modern Scenario

Today, new substances go through this process of proving, and add to homoeopathic remedies available. Hippocrates wrote, "By similar things a disease is produced and through the application of the like it is cured."

People are often familiar with medicines that suppress symptoms, that actually harm the cells in the body, and have other definite negative chemical or physical reaction on the body. Homoeopathy seeks to repel the imbalance from the body and allow the body to heal and rebalance. Homoeopathy stimulates the body's natural curative powers. Homoeopaths therefore choose a remedy based on provings and the homoeopathic 'Law of Similars' (and not a chemical or suppressive action).

Nowadays, homoeopathy focuses more on the psychological symptoms, while in older days the emphasis was on the physical expression of disease. This has led to the system of dream provings. In a dream proving the healthy volunteer lays the test remedy under the pillow. In this type of proving homoeopathy works with higher potentiated remedies. The energy of the remedy will cause certain dreams, very different from the dreams the volunteer usually has. Often these proving dreams are filled with symbolic images and clues related to the character of the remedy. These provings may shed more light on the mental and emotional symptoms, but they are also much more difficult to interpret. Provings are now mostly conducted by students of homoeopathy, and there are now more provings of a very high standard than there have been proved in the last few years and have become important remedies that have helped many patients to a higher level of health.

Since Hahnemann first made the proving of quinine thousands of provings have been carried out by homoeopaths and their volunteers. All remedies are tested on humans. Poisonings (or accidental provings) have provided another source of valuable information to homoeopathy, substances such as deadly nightshade (Belladonna) and snake venoms and many others are of tremendous value.

Homoeopathy is a dynamic medicine, and volunteers continue to prove new remedies on a regular basis. There are many *Materia Medicas* used by homoeopaths today. The remedy name is followed by proving symptoms. The categories are similar in each, starting with mind symptoms, head, face and down to the various systems in the body, the extremities, etc. When wanting to look up a particular symptom and the possible remedies which have shown that symptom under provings, homoeopaths look in repertories. The descriptive way to write the symptoms are called rubrics. These rubrics are also listed in the same similar order in repertories.

There is no doubt that more and more people will add to the list of the provings, for whatever Hahnemann postulated in *The Organon* have come true as scientific facts.

Commonly Asked Questions

1. Why should anyone go to a homoeopathic doctor?

Homoeopathic treatment is suitable for most people, and has the advantage of being completely safe when used correctly. A homoeopath makes efforts to see the disease holistically, and that is the main reason why this system is getting more acceptability.

2. Are homoeopathic medicines safe for children?

Yes, they can be given safely to even the youngest infant.

3. How are homoeopathic remedies prepared?

Homoeopathic remedies are prepared by grinding the active ingredient, and mixing it with alcohol and water, then allowing it to soften and steep. The mixture is then filtered to produce what is called a tincture, made more potent by dilution, which increases the healing power while decreasing the concentration.

There are many different potency ranges. The best tincture has a potency of 1x. To make a 2x potency, one part of the base is mixed with nine parts alcohol, and shaken ten times. To make a 3x potency, one part of 2x potency is mixed with nine parts alcohol and shaken again. This process is continued until the desired dilution is acquired. In addition to alcohol, other mixing agents include water, glycerine and lactose.

Homoeopathic medicines come in C potencies as well as X potencies. There are k potencies as well. The 1000 k potency is labelled as 1m, a 10,000k potency as 10m, and so on.

Homoeopathic doctors prescribe their remedies in pellets, tablets and dilutions (liquids). The mixing, or potentiation, affects the way a homoeopathic medicine works. In general, the lower potencies, like 3x and 6x, have a larger effect, and are used for acute illnesses, and are taken once every 15 minutes to once every four hours. Medium potencies, like 12x and 30x, affect the senses and nervous system, and are used for chronic conditions. They are taken once a day to three times a day. High potencies, like 60x and above, affect mental conditions, and are taken once a month to once a year.

4. Do homoeopathic medicines have any side effects?

Homoeopathic medicines have no side effects. The term 'side effects' of a medicine comes from modern pharmacology. These drugs are aimed at one area of the body, such as the cardiovascular system, the gut, the kidneys, etc. Though they have a primary area of action, they also affect other areas of the body. If these effects are undesirable, they are known as adverse side effects. Homoeopathic medicines are not employed against one particular area or organ of the body. The homoeopathic remedy is chosen because it matches as closely as possible with the totality of symptoms of the patient. Side effects, such as tissue destruction, do not occur under homoeopathy.

5. Can homoeopathic medicines be taken safely during pregnancy?

The safety of homoeopathic medicines is well known. Still, it is advisable to take the opinion of a homoeopathic doctor in such a situation.

6. Who can take homoeopathy treatment? Do you have to be sick, old, young, healthy?

No, as with all healing, homoeopathy depends on the body's vitality. If the overall vitality is very low, the best plan might be to take it slowly with lower potencies, and work step by step. Even if you feel very healthy, you can work on what is called a 'constitutional' plan—usually with a homoeopath—to find the remedy which suits you best mentally and physically. In between, you are never too young, too old or too in-between to benefit from homoeopathy's many healing solutions.

7. Can homoeopathic remedies cure acute symptoms and personal concerns?

Homoeopathic remedies, correctly chosen, are capable of affecting cure for acute symptoms as well as deep personal cures. Arsenic, for example, can cause symptoms which we could easily relate to food poisoning: severe vomiting, diarrhoea—but the homoeopathic dilution of arsenic, *Arsenicum alb*, when taken for acute stomach flu or food poisoning, brings much relief, both during and after the necessary purging, minimising discomfort and recovery time. If you were to take arsenic in small poisonings over a longer time, you would likely become very restless, especially at night, irritable with weakness and exhaustion; you would move constantly, grow very afraid of death, being left along, and might even become suicidal, miserly, selfish and malicious.

Thus with higher potencies and professional guidance, you can use *Arsenicum alb* to treat individuals whose lives have somehow driven them to similar despair. The remedies really can resonate that deeply, but at least at this level of care, the remedy selection and dosage is critical. Just as certain things in nature can, in susceptible individuals, cause hay fever, constipation, headaches, rashes, pains and so on, those very things can stimulate healing responses, both acute and manifest.

8. Are homoeopathic medicines compatible with one's other medicines?

Homoeopathy is 100 per cent compatible with other medications. That is, it will not interfere with the effectiveness of other medicines. It is possible that other medicines will lessen the effectiveness of homoeopathy. Depending on the patient's sensitivity, many remedies can be antidoted by strong odours, steroidal medicines, caffeine or even homoeopathic remedies.

Higher potencies, used in constitutional therapy, are more sensitive to antidoting, especially in the first day or two after dosing. There are a few remedies that should never be taken together, especially in high potency *Apis* and *Rhus tox*.

9. What will one's homoeopath need to know?

In order to find the right remedy for you as an individual, your homoeopath will need to know all about you. A detailed understanding of who you are, along with any complaints and details of how you experience them, is needed to assess your case correctly. So anything you can tell your homoeopath that is typical of who you are will help this process. Finding out about your general energy level, your past medical history and the way you live are also important. Anything you say will be treated in the strictest confidence. The initial consultation may last an hour or more.

10. Is it a fact that homoeopathy is too slow as a system of treatment?

Causes of acute diseases or disorders, like headache, fever, cold, cough, etc., can be cured within minutes through the proper selection of the homoeopathic remedy. However, chronic diseases like asthma, heart problems, cancer, etc., need time to cure.

There is a belief that allopathic medicines give immediate relief, but at what cost? The use of strong medicines and steroids weaken the body's natural immune system. Homoeopathy restores the body to its original state of health. If a disease is chronic in nature it means that it would have been in the human body for a long time, so it requires some time to be cured. This can vary depending on the problem and the patient.

Generally, a strict diet is required while taking homoeopathic medicines. Stimulants like coffee, strong tea, nicotine, alcohol, etc., must be avoided as far as possible as they interfere with the working of the medicine, and the healing process slows down.

There are numerous cases of long-standing diseases and of serious nature, like kidney failure, heart problems, severe asthma, which have been cured within a few days.

11. Can homoeopathy treat anything and everything?

Like any other systems of medicine, homoeopathy has its own limitations. Through homoeopathy, any ailment, acute or chronic, local or general, can be treated except diseases where surgery is unavoidable. Some of the so-called surgical problems, like enlarged tonsils, sinusitis, piles, fistula, kidney stone, etc., in the early stages can be treated with homoeopathic medicines to a large extent.

12. How does homoeopathy remedy work?

Homoeopathic remedies work by stimulating the body's own healing power. This stimulus will assist your own system to clear itself of any expressions of imbalance. The aim is to get you to a level of health so that eventually you will need infrequent treatment.

13. What will the treatment be like?

Your homoeopath will give you a homoeopathic remedy, usually in the form of a tablet or tablets, occasionally as powders, which should be allowed to dissolve in your mouth; or you may be given a liquid remedy with instructions. Nothing else should be put in the mouth for half an hour before or after taking the medicine, not even toothpaste or cigarette. Your homoeopath will usually advise you to avoid strong intakes, like coffee or tea, peppermint, and preparations containing menthol, eucalyptus and camphor, as these can interfere with the action of the homoeopathic remedy. Do make sure that you understand the instructions before you leave.

14. What will happen once treatment starts?

After taking your remedy you may notice some changes. Some patients experience a period of exceptional well-being and optimism. Sometimes your symptoms can appear to get worse for a short time. This is a good sign that the remedy is taking effect. Sometimes, a cold, rash or some form of discharge may appear as a spring-cleaning effect which means your system is going through a clearing out stage.

Similarly, old symptoms can reappear, usually for a short period. These symptoms will pass, and must not be treated as they are a very important part of the healing process. If any response to your treatment concerns you, do contact your homoeopath as soon as you can, as treatment progresses. You might also want to make notes of any changes, and take them with you to discuss at your next appointment.

16. How long does the treatment take?

This depends very much on what sort of illness you have, as well as the other individual characteristics of your case, So, it is not realistic for your homoeopath to assess this until it can be seen how you respond to the remedies prescribed over some time. It is possible to say that a slowly developing complaint, or one that has been experienced for some years, will not disappear immediately although there may be a response and some improvement quite soon. Other acute complaints may get better quickly.

Homoeopathy cures from the inside, and often outer symptoms, such as a skin complaint, are the last to clear. Be patient! In the long term it is much better for you to be cured of both the cause of your illness and its symptoms, rather than merely relieving or suppressing the symptoms. Remember that every case is different, and no two patients are alike.

15. What ailments can be treated by homoeopathy?

Almost all ailments are amenable to homoeo treatment. But homoeopathy is best known for its ability to treat chronic ailments. The reason for this that homoeopathy is the only system of medicine which offers curative treatment (not palliative) in many chronic ailments which have been declared incurable by other schools of medicine. Be it skin disease, chronic gastric and intestinal disorders, chronic fatigue syndrome, migraine, asthama, allergic disorders, arthritis, psychological disorders, etc., all these and many more chronic ailments have been affected curatively by homoeopathy. The only major limiting factors are:

a. Gross structural and pathological changes.

b. Very low vitality of the patient.

c. Unavoidable presence of certain causative or maintaining factors.

Then homoeopathy is also known to make surgery on many occasions. Many tonsils, adenoids, appendices, etc., have been saved with homoeopathy. Benign tumours and renal stones also respond well to homoeopathic treatment. Even in case where curative treatment is not possible, like advanced cases of arthritis, malignancies, etc., management and palliation with homoeopathic medicines is very effective, and improves the quality of life of such patients without making them suffer the side effects of the modern wonder drugs.

Homoeopathy is also very effective in acute ailments. And the action of a rightly selected medicine is usually faster than any other medicines. Not only this, under proper homoeopathic treatment, the tendency to frequent recurrence of acutes and their tendency to become chronic is aborted.

17. How can there be any physiological effect if homoeopaths use such small doses of medicine?

Although we don't understand precisely how homoeopathic medicines work, there is clear evidence that the medicines are active and can heal. Homoeopathy became popular in the US and Europe during the 1800's because of its success in treating the many infectious diseases that raged during that time, including yellow fever, scarlet fever, cholera and many others. The death rate in homoeopathic hospitals was between one-half to one-eight of those in conventional medical hospitals. Homoeopathic medicines also have been shown to work on infants and on various animals (including dogs, cats, horses and even cows) where it is highly unlikely that they are acting only as a placebo.

Homoeopaths also find that people who are being treated with homoeopathic medicine for a chronic disease sometimes experience a temporary exacerbation in their symptoms as the body's defences are being stimulated. They have found that a healing crisis is sometimes necessary to achieve healing. It is highly unlikely that this temporary worsening of symptoms is the result of a placebo response.

There has also been some good scientific research published in medical journals and other scientific publications. *The Lancet* (September 20, 1997) published a review of 89 double-blind or randomised placebo-controlled clinical trials. The authors conclude that the clinical effects of homoeopathic medicines are not simply the results of placebo. In fact, they found that homoeopathic medicines had nearly three times greater effect than placebo. Another research in a British journal indicated that there had been 107 controlled clinical trials, 81 of which showed that the homoeopathic medicines had beneficial results. It is important to know that the small doses used by homoeopaths only have an effect when a person has a hypersensitivity to the small doses given. If the wrong medicine is given to a person, nothing happens. If the correct medicine is given, the medicine acts as a catalyst to the person's defences. In any case, homoeopathic medicines do not have side effects.

18. How must the homoeopathic medicines be stored?

In a dry place, away from the sun, and strong perfumes. Not in the refrigerator.

19. What is the difference between homoeopathy and herbs?

Herbs are considered natural substances, but they differ greatly from homoeopathic remedies. Like traditional Western medicine, herbs are complex substances that need to be broken down inside the body before they can be used by cells. This conversion requires energy. Homoeopathic remedies, because of the way they are prepared, are simple medicines that are readily used by cells, even by the cells of those who are very sick. Since homoeopathic medicines come in such highly diluted concentrations, it is extremely unlikely that they will cause side effects or toxic reactions. This is not so with herbs. Herbs may cause side effects, allergic or toxic reactions, like traditional Western drugs.

20. How does the concept of homoeopathy differ from that of conventional medicine?

Homoeopathy attempts to stimulate the body to heal itself. First, we must accept that all symptoms, no matter how uncomfortable they are, represent the body's attempt to restore itself to health. Instead of looking upon the symptoms as something wrong which must be set right, we see them as signs of the way the body is attempting to help itself. Instead of looking upon the symptoms as something wrong which must be set right, we see them as signs of the way the body is attempting to help itself. Instead of trying to stop the cough with suppressants, as conventional medicine does, a homoeopath will give a remedy that will cause a cough in a healthy person, and does stimulate the ill body to restore itself.

Second, we must look at the totality of the symptoms presented. We each experience a cough in our unique way. Yet conventional medicine acts as if all coughs were alike. It, therefore, offers a series of suppressive drugs—something to suppress the cough, something to dry the mucus, something to lower the histamine level, something to ease falling asleep. Homoeopathy, on the other hand, looks for the one substance that will cause similar symptoms in a healthy person. In conventional medicine, health is seen simply as the absence of the disease. To a homoeopath, health is much more. A healthy person is one who is free on all levels—physical, emotional and mental.

21. What if my child or I have food or environmental allergies?

Homoeopathy treats the whole person. When you are given a homoeopathic medicine that closely matches your symptoms and states, you will experience greater energy and vitality, and your immune system will become stronger. It is typical for patients who respond well to homoeopathy to be able to go back to eating or being exposed to substances that bothered them prior to homoeopathic treatment.

22. Are there any preventive medicines in homoeopathy?

Usually a patient on constitutional medicine does not develop any illness, and enjoys good health. Apart from any other specific medicine to an illness constitutional medicine is the best preventive medicine. At times it has been seen that a specific medicine for example, *Euphrasia* taken for conjunctivitis, precipitates the illness rather than stimulating it. For the same reason, it is advisable to take constitutional treatment as a preventive treatment instead of a specific medicine.

23. Is it safe to use homoeopathic medicines while one is breastfeeding or pregnant?

Yes. Homoeopathic medicines are safe, and do not have the toxic side effects of many allopathic medicines, making homoeopathy an excellent choice of medicine during pregnancy and breastfeeding. Women are grateful to know that they can seek relief from the pain, for example, of mastitis or haemorrhoids, without harming themselves or their babies.

24. Do homoeopathic medicines have any expiration date?

Yes. Although not required by law, homoeopathic manufacturers place expiration dates on their remedies because of guidelines set forth by the Homoeopathic Pharmacopoeia. But if kept away from radiation (electromagnetic), heat and light, remedies have shown to be effective 10-20 years after their noted expiration date (normally about 3-5 years).

25. Can someone who is lactose intolerant or diabetic take homoeopathic remedies?

The amount of milk sugar (lactose) and/or sucrose that would be taken is minimal. Homoeopathic remedies are not taken every day for a long period of time. If there is still concern in taking the remedy, it can be diluted in water and taken that way.

26. How does homoeopathy differ from herbal medicine, naturopathy and acupuncture?

While homoeopathy and these healing arts are similar in that they do not employ drugs or other conventional medicinal procedures, each one is also quite distinctive. Naturopathy is a broad term encompassing a host of natural healing arts ranging from nutrition to water cures. Acupuncture is one branch of Oriental medicine that stimulates and balances the body's energy. Herbal medicine, also known as 'botanical medicine', uses material doses of plant substances for treatment. Homoeopathy is generally considered a natural healing art. It does not originate in the Orient, nor does it use material doses of substances.

27. What is classical homoeopathy, and how does it differ from modern homoeopathy?

Classical homoeopathy is the type taught by its founder, Dr Samuel Hahnemann, who claimed that at any given time only one remedy should be given to the patient, the one that has the greatest similarity to his disease. This process of finding the correct remedy is very tedious, and requires a lot of search on the part of the physician. But if it is found, the therapeutic results are impressive and satisfying. If this unique remedy cannot be found for this patient the results are from zero to a small amelioration of the condition. So many homoeopaths who do not know what remedy to prescribe, or do not have the time to take a proper case, and search and study it, they may give three, four or up to 20 remedies hoping that the right one would be within these remedies. This is a type of homoeopathy that is not classical, and, of course, does not give the result, that the correct remedy should have given.

28. What are the sources from which homoeopathic remedies are derived?

Homoeopathic remedies are derived from raw, natural sources, generally from the animal, vegetable or mineral kingdoms.

29. What works better—liquids or pills?

They are both equally effective. Pills are dissolved under the tongue, and the remedy is absorbed via the sublingual tissues. This allows the remedy to begin its work faster than if they were swallowed.

30. What is the difference between an X and a C potency?

An x potency is diluted on a 1:9 scale, that is one part substance to nine parts liquid. A C potency is diluted on a scale of 1:99, that is, one part substance to 99 parts liquid. Therefore, a C potency, by being more dilute, may be considered 'stronger' homoeopathically. However, stronger is not always better. If you wanted a 30C but can only get a 30x, the latter would be fine because both have been diluted 30 times. It is the correct remedy, not the potency, that makes the difference.

31. How many pills are in a dose?

Each manufacturer determines the dose for its remedies. This can vary from 1 pill to 10 pills. It is recommended to take 3 to 5 pills, no matter what the pill size. Your homoeopath may also tell you how many pills to take and, in that instance, be sure you follow your doctor's directions.

32. Why is homoeopathy so popular?

Homoeopathic treatment works with your body's own healing powers to bring health and well-being. Patients are treated as individuals, not as a collection of disease labels. Homoeopathy treats all your symptoms—mental, emotional and physical. Homoeopathic remedies are gentle, subtle and powerful.

33. Is homoeopathy the same as vaccination?

The law of similars (that which makes one sick shall also heal) principle of homoeopathy is often compared to vaccination. Vaccine introduces a small amount of the weakened virus or bacterium related to a disease into the body in order to raise the body's immune response against that disease. However, homoeopathy is quite different because homoeopathic remedies are extremely diluted, and therefore no diseased material (biological or chemical trace) is introduced into the body.

Another fundamental difference is that a homoeopathic prescription is specific to that particular patient, and stimulates the body's immune system to be strengthened against all illness, not just a single disease.

34. What are self-healing powers?

Since medicine began, it has been recognised that there is a capacity for self-healing within the human organism. In acute illnesses, such as colds, chickenpox, etc., the body naturally resists infection, and, in time, gets better through mobilising its own defences, helped by rest, fresh air and the right food. In more long-lasting chronic illnesses, such as repeated migraine or depression, the body's vitality is often too depleted to do this without assistance. In these cases, the right remedy will stimulate the body's self-healing powers to start the process of cure.

Over many years this self-healing power has been given various names in different cultures—prana in India, *chi* in China, and vital force in Europe. Researchers have attempted to localise it in what is called, in modern medical terminology, the immune system. It is not yet completely clear to anyone what exactly it is in us that heals disease, though we often see demonstrations of its power.

35. Can animals be treated with homoeopathy?

Homoeopathy is as effective for animals as it is for humans.

36. What is constitutional treatment in homoeopathy?

Although Hahnemann himself did not have an explicit theory of physical constitution or psychological dispositions, he did observe that general symptoms pertaining to the whole organism (for example, reactions to weather, perspiration and sleep patterns) plus the patient's disposition were of special importance both diagnostically and for case management. Later homoeopaths, notably James Tyler Kent, increasingly used overall disposition as a basis for determining the remedy and assessing the patient's vitality in response to treatment. Such treatment, which was applied in cases of chronic illness, became known as constitutional prescribing. Recent developments in the understanding of remedies and the homoeopathic process, such as George Vithoulkas's essence prescribing, and Rajan Sankaran's concept of central delusion are continuation of this trend.

Since in the present social context classical homoeopaths are usually seen for chronic complaints, these principles feature prominently in current homoeopathic education and practice. In accordance with this view of disease, classical homoeopathic treatment of chronic disease requires a long interview, often longer than an hour, to determine the totality of the patient's symptoms: a thorough history is taken, including childhood and physically or psychologically traumatic or memorable events; important or recurrent dreams are elicited; and a unified understanding of the person's unique perception of the world is sought.

37. Why are miasms so difficult to understand?

Although nowadays homoeopathy is especially known for its treatment of chronic diseases, Hahnemann recognised already early on that homoeopathy, like conventional medicine, had more difficulty with these than with acute illnesses. In response, in his later years, he developed the concept of miasms, an idea that is still as complex as it ever was, and which remains contentious. After some years of homoeopathic experience he began noticing that many of his chronic patients tended to relapse even after prolonged homoeopathic treatment. Though they responded to remedies, over time their symptoms would tend to shift around without a fundamental improvement in their state. This led to his hypothesising that health was not only determined by the person's present vitality, but also related to historical factors in the person's own life, as well as that of immediate ancestors, what he called *miasm* (from the Greek for 'taint'). These factors had to be addressed before the patient could experience satisfactory improvement of the symptoms, while in cases where the miasmatic load was heavy, only partial improvement was to be expected.

Hahnemann described three types of miasms in his *The Chronic Disease:*

a. *Psora* (possibly from Greek for 'itch'): This was associated with cutaneous manifestations such as scabies, as well as diseases that tended to present as constantly irritating or distracting, yet completely reversible (for example, eczema, mild asthma, recurring infections). Hahnemann considered this the primordial miasm, arguing that improper treatment of such manifestations throughout history was what led to chronic disease and other miasms.

b. *Sycosis* (from the Greek for fig-wart): This was associated with genital infections such as fig-wart and gonorrhoea. These infections and diseases such as cutaneous warts, benign tumours and psychological neuroses had the shared quality of being relatively fixed yet non-life-threatening. Psychologically such states were associated with the need to accept the problem as an irremediable defect.

c. *Syphilis* (from the disease name), was associated with syphilis and other manifestations such as bone ulcers, organic heart disease, and dementia that had the shared tendency of producing irreversible tissue destruction.

Later in the nineteenth century the following miasms, which are considered immediate in severity between sycosis and syphilis, were further delineated:

d. *Tuberculosis:* Associated with the infection as well as life-threatening yet reversible asthma or pneumonia and (psychologically) with constant dissatisfaction and the desire for change.

e. *Cancer:* Associated with malignant states as well as obsessive-compulsive desire and psychological traits of perfectionism, and excessive responsibility or ambition.

More recently, the highly influential Raja Sankaran has further developed the understanding of the psychological qualities of miasms, and has made miasms an integral aspect of his diagnostic approach. He further expanded the list of miasm by largely supplanting psora in favour of several, more specific miasms, previously subsumed under it:

a. *Acute:* Diseases (whether acute or chronic) that present with a pattern of recovery (with no ill effects) or succumb.

b. *Typhus:* (after the clinical pattern of the infection): Enormous, short-term struggle followed by recovery.

c. *Ringworm:* (after the clinical pattern of the infection): Cyclical recovery followed by likely recurrence.

d. *Malaria:* (after the clinical pattern of the infection): Low-grade, fixed illness (similar to a sycotic manifestation) punctuated by acute exacerbations.

He further added a miasm between cancer and syphilis:

e. *Leprosy:* (after the clinical pattern of the infection): Destructive, irreversible, yet not necessarily life-threatening manifestations such as leprosy and other disfigurements and AIDS that lead to both physical and social disability.

Miasms are determined through careful inquiry into the patient's personal and family medical history in search for previous infections (especially ones that from which recovery was incomplete) such as tuberculosis or diseases such as cancer. The presence of such manifestation can influence the choice of remedy beyond the presenting symptoms, and also provides a prognostic measure in a similar way as familial inheritance influences prognosis in conventional medicine.

The acceptance of miasms varies within the homoeopathic community. Some homoeopaths find the concept unhelpful or otherwise unacceptable; others will make occasional use of it; while yet others strive in every case to determine the miasmatic nature of the illness in order to facilitate prescribing (since remedy selection can be assisted by knowledge of the miasm). Of the latter two groups some regard miasms as objective features of the disease, while others view them merely as clinically useful categorisations.

Understanding miasms will probably always be somewhat difficult but time, study and experience will establish a proper foundation. At least, then it will feel more comfortable to use the miasmatic theory. This is especially true when many well-selected remedies have proven ineffective and temporary. The difficulty lies in the complex nature of the diseased state and the subsequent reactions of the human system.

38. If homoeopathy is so effective, why has it not overtaken allopathy.

Whatever criteria you may use, there is no doubt that homoeopathy is much more effective than allopathy, but the sad fact is that homoeopathy has lagged behind in popularity. The failure is not of the system, but of the physician. Homoeopathy is a science and has its principles which have to be properly applied to find the right remedy (the *similimum*). Homoeopathy has more than 2,000 remedies to choose from. Even if you filter out the not-so-used ones, you get more than 200 remedies. Choosing one among them is not so easy and requires the application of great skills on the part of the physician. Also, the homoeopathic colleges have totally failed in teaching homoeopathy as per the principles laid down by Hahnemann. This has resulted in doctors prescribing compound drugs (which is prohibited by Hahnemann, who calls for only one remedy to be prescribed at a time). Thus, their treatment is a hit-and-run affair. A number of homoeopaths who neither understand nor are able to apply this treatment, prescribe allopathic medicines and thus discredit homoeopathy. In fact, the number of doctors who properly apply the scientific principles of homoeopathy are but a few. This is the only reason why homoeopathy has not overtaken allopathy. To quote Mahatma Gandhi, "Just like my principle of ahimsa (non-violence) homeopathy can never fail. Failure, if any, is the person who practises it."

39. Can homoeopathy be practised by anyone?

The answer to this is, yes. Anyone who has truly understood the principle of *Simplex, Similimum, Minimum* and anyone who is committed to the system of holistic healing, can practise homoeopathy even if they are not certified doctors. What is required is a knowledge of biology, knowledge of the human anatomy and physiology, and most importantly, the knowledge of symptomatology, that is, diseases and their symptoms. This knowledge coupled with the mastery over the principles and a thorough understanding of the *Materia Medica* will help in the practice of homoeopathy. However, it is a fallacy that homoeopathy can be practised by reading books, but by understanding and applying principles homoeopathy can be practised.

40. What are the different types of medicines used in homoeopathy?

Homoeopathy uses an array of medicines whose source ranges from animals to plants and chemicals. Plants like onion, capsicum, belladonna, cactus, etc., are used for preparation of homoeopathic medicines. A large number of chemicals like nitric acid, iron, phosphorus are popular homoeopathic remedies. There are also a large number of animal-sourced medicines which are snake poisons. Medicines are also prepared from substances like milk and sand. The products of diseases are used to prepare homoeopathic medicines called *nosodes*. These nosodes include carsinocin (prepared from the cancer cells), and tuberculinum (prepared from the cells of the lungs of cow infected by tuberculosis), etc. While there may be a few people who are apprehensive of taking such medicines, they need not fear, because the process of preparing homoeopathic medicines ensures that they are diluted such that they lose their original form, and are rendered harmless.

41. Is there any diet restriction while taking homoeopathic medicines? Any advice on lifestyle?

It is a myth regarding restrictions in diet, like onion, garlic, *paan,* tobacco, or using perfumes. These medicines have been successfully used on patients who are habituated to coffee and betel leaves. These medicines always act. But some restrictions are advised with certain medicines only, for there is the possibility of their action being nullified. But as a general precautionary measure, it is always better to avoid using anything that is strong. A homoeopath may suggest changes if it seems that this is contributing to one's illness, of course, a good basic diet is necessary for good health, with less sugars, fats, alcohol and refined foods. There is an increasing awareness of the benefits of foods free from artificial colourings, preservatives and flavourings. Whole foods and organic foods, free from chemicals, pesticides and fertilisers, are also increasingly available.

42. What is a trituration?

This is a remedy made in lactose (milk sugar). The substance is ground for hours, using a pestle and mortar. The powder, or triturate, can then be formed into tablets.

43. Are all remedies available in liquid?

No, this is due to the nature of the substance that is being made into a remedy. For example, gold (aurum metallicum) is not soluble in water or alcohol until it has been triturated to the 8x potency (4C). At this potency level, it can then be converted to a liquid and then sold at a 10x or a 4c dilution in liquid to be available in dilution form.

44. What are the short-term and long-term benefits of homoeopathy?

The short-term benefits of using homoeopathy are: minimising effect, avoiding suppression, preserving strength, minimising healing/recovery time. Often the first benefit one receives from the remedy is the localisation of symptoms; the second level of benefits is more curative. For example, you know how even a badly stubbed toe or pinched finger can upset your applecart, keeping you from thinking of anything else? The first thing you notice after a dose of *Hypericum* is that the toe is just a toe again, though still a sore one; that's half the battle. The next half, the actual easing of pain and tenderness follows soon after (especially if you have *Arnica* to control bruising). If you actually broke your toe, *Hypericum* would not numb the pain to the point that you would not realise it was in a crisis. The same rule applies to emotional symptoms. With *Ignatia*, grief, for example, is not cloaked to the point that you have to re-experience the news every four to six hours. But it can give you enough distance to find your strength between waves of grief and disbelief, and can also prevent suppression, thus making the most of a sad situation. Food poisoning/stomach flu can have similar results. Since it will not suppress the necessary purging, *Ars alb* (or the indicated remedy) can give great comfort to those awful restless intervals between vomiting, plus relieve much of the colic and discomfort of purging as also offer the most efficient cleansing available.

The long-term benefits of using homoeopathy are lowered susceptibility via a stronger immune system and a greater sense of balance, especially when reaping the benefits of professional constitutional care. That is, remedy work that goes beyond temporary or nagging symptoms to balancing the whole picture— mentally, emotionally and physically. Wouldn't it be great to be in that percentile that did not get last year's flu or your regular hay fever, migraine or arthritis? The same susceptibility applies to emotions. Wouldn't it be great to always rise above a situation instead of ending up feeling insulted, jealous or unduly hurt? Homoeopathy leaves your system stronger, not weaker, and certainly better at tackling life's next hurdle—safe and effective system of medicine that helps the body's efforts to heal itself by dosing it with minute potentised quantities of the plant, mineral or animal by-product capable (in full strength) of creating similar symptoms to those presented by the patient.